District Nursing

To Miss E.M. Wearn, Teacher and Friend

District Nursing

Margaret Illing

BA, SRN, SCM, QIDNS, HV Cert., District Nurse Tutor

Member of the Council for the Education and Training of Health Visitors and part-time District Nurse Tutor, Brighton Polytechnic; previously Head of the Department of Applied Social Studies, Croydon College, London

Brian Donovan

BSc, MSc, MA

Senior Lecturer in Sociology and Social Administration, Croydon College, London

Foreword by

Lisbeth Hockey, OBE, PhD, FRCN
Director, Nursing Research Unit,
University of Edinburgh

BAILLIÈRE TINDALL · LONDON

A BAILLIÈRE TINDALL book published by
Cassell Ltd,
35 Red Lion Square, London WC1R 4SG

and at Sydney, Toronto

an affiliate of
Macmillan Publishing Co. Inc.
New York

First published 1981

ISBN 0 7020 0878 8

Typeset by Inforum Ltd, Portsmouth
Printed and bound in Great Britain
by Billing and Sons Limited
Guildford, London, Oxford, Worcester

British Library Cataloguing in Publication Data

Illing, Margaret
   District nursing.
   1. Community health nursing
   I. Title   II. Donovan, Brian
   610.73'4   RT98

   ISBN 0-7020-0878-8

Contributors

Ivy Price, SRN, SCM, QIDNS, HV Cert., HV Tutor's Certificate, DN Tutor, *Principal Lecturer in District Nursing, West London Institute of Higher Education*

Ruth Sharman, BA, SRN, SCM, NDN Cert., HV Cert., CHNT Cert., HV Tutor, *DN Tutor, Institute of Advanced Nursing Education*

Contents

> *The historical context* – home care before the National Health
> Service – the statutory service – the inquiries of the fifties and
> subsequent change. *The development of the concept of primary
> health care* – teamwork in primary care – hospital liaison
> schemes – the growth of the night nursing service – the
> nursing team and the concept of support. *Research into the
> district nursing service* – changes in the attitude to training
> – the extended role of the district nurse. *Basic ideas and values*
> – comprehensive patient care – continuity of care – the
> containment of disease.

SECTION ONE – THE PROFESSIONAL SKILLS

> *Identification of problems* – the goals of care. *The nursing history
> and framework for assessment* – the head-to-toe body systems
> approach – fundamental human needs – referral of patients to
> the district nurse – initial relationships. *The patient and
> family interview* – defining the problem. *Aims, goals and plans
> of care* – advantages of the process in caseload management.

> *Caseload management* – how patients come into domiciliary
> care – the first visit. *Frequency of visiting* – duration of
> dependency. *The care of drugs. Problems experienced by certain
> patients* – child patients – patients suffering from cancer –
> helping the bereaved – elderly patients – the isolated patient.
> *Maintaining standards of care. The management of change.*

SECTION TWO – THE HEALTH AND SOCIAL CONTEXT

Foreword

I consider it a privilege to have been invited to write the foreword for this book, which will meet an urgent need. While texts to help learners in their basic preparation for nursing and in many nursing specialties have proliferated over the past few years, district nursing appears to have been bypassed, thus leaving a serious gap in the nursing literature.

Margaret Illing has responded to the challenge of filling this gap. Her rich experience is reflected in a book which captures the complexity of district nursing. In tracing the development of professional awareness and sketching the contemporary legislative and administrative framework, the authors succeed well in giving district nursing its proper place in the total spectrum of health and welfare services. The skills of district nursing identified in the text give ample support to the introduction of mandatory training for this developing and important nursing specialty.

Future learners are particularly fortunate in having access to this book, but it will also be helpful to qualified nurses whose work is related to district nursing, be it education, administration or direct patient care.

June, 1981   *Lisbeth Hockey*

Preface

The authors of this book, three tutors and a teacher of social policy, have been aware for some time of the need for a new textbook on district nursing. The students need an introduction to some of the perspectives through which their work may be studied, and this need will be more urgent when they enter the new extended course before they start to practise.

This book is derived from research studies and the practical experiences of both authors and students. We have discussed our ideas in the classroom, asked students and practical work teachers to report back findings from practice and, together with colleagues from both service and education, we have evolved some simple principles. These enjoyable exchanges have sometimes provoked fierce argument and, over the years, we have been aware of considerable shifts in our thinking.

The reader will recognise that this book is a background to the teaching and practical experience on a course. Some further reading will be suggested by the references at the end of each chapter. Learning about district nursing is like travelling through a forest. There are many paths, some more suitable than others, and this book provides a signpost. Throughout we have provided guidelines and suggestions that will help the student starting practical work, but we have not disguised the complexity of the decisions she will have to make either alone or with her colleagues in the primary health care team.

As in many nursing textbooks, for clarity and convenience, we have referred to all district nurses and patients' relatives as women and to all patients as men. We know this will not be taken amiss by our male colleagues whose contribution to district nursing is both well-known and well-respected.

This book is dedicated to Miss E.M. Wearn who from 1943–1957 was District Nursing Superintendent at the Lady Rayleigh Training Home at Leytonstone in Essex. In 1949 I was one of her students and once qualified I stayed on her staff. From Miss Wearn I learned about domiciliary patient care, professional practice and much, much more besides.

June, 1981   *Margaret Illing*

Acknowledgements

The idea of this book arose from our work at Croydon College and our debt is primarily to our colleagues there, our students and their practical work teachers. I am grateful to all my friends and colleagues in the district nursing service who have helped me distil my ideas into a form that I hope is useful.

Grateful acknowledgement for permission to reproduce material is made as follows:

To the Nursing Times for material from *Nursing Outlook*, 9 November, 1978, on care of the stroke patient. To the Queen's Nursing Institute for material from their handbook *Training for Independence*, and for material regarding the regulations for the holding and disposal of scheduled drugs reproduced from *District Nursing*, November 1963.

I am particularly grateful to Lisbeth Hockey and Ivy Price for their criticism and advice, and to Julie Trangmar, who shared with me her teaching notes on communication. To Rose Baker for her help and encouragement, and Shirley Knight who typed and retyped the manuscript.

CHAPTER 1

The Development of Professional Awareness

THE HISTORICAL CONTEXT

Much has been written about the origins of district nursing[1], but it is to the recent past that we must look for clues as to why the beliefs and values held today have developed. One of the most significant events was the implementation of the National Health Service Act in 1948 when district nursing became a statutory service.

HOME CARE BEFORE THE NATIONAL HEALTH SERVICE

In the first half of the twentieth century the hospital service comprised the voluntary hospitals, the workhouses, isolation hospitals and asylums. Even in those days they were inadequate for their purpose as medical science was developing and treatments were replacing the often begrudging care of the nineteenth century. Home care was available to patients who were able to pay fees to their general practitioners and to those who were insured through membership of a trade union or a friendly society. The National Health Insurance Act 1911 had made it compulsory for low paid workers to be insured, but in all cases benefits were only available to the wage earner. Wives, children, the aged, the disabled and the handicapped were without access to free medical care at home, and had to pay the general practitioner's fee or rely upon the outpatient departments of the voluntary hospitals or dispensaries run by charities.

Home nursing was provided by nurses employed by voluntary nursing associations throughout the country. This service was financed by a scheme of weekly payments made by the residents of the neighbourhood supplemented by such fund raising activities as flag days, sales of work and whist drives, together with payments made on behalf of patients by some friendly societies, some employers, and for the very poor by the public assistance. Patients not covered by any insurance were required to pay for their treatment, or at least pay as much as they were able. Collecting subscriptions was an irksome chore for district nurses, and estimating how much a patient who was not insured should pay was a difficult and often distasteful task complicating the assessment of nursing need. Many nurses preferred to care for patients who could not afford to pay at all rather than have to ask for money at each visit.

To avoid patients consulting the nurse rather than the doctor, whose consulting fees were higher than the payment to the voluntary association, the nurse was forbidden to visit a patient who was not receiving care from their doctor. If the nurse was called by the patient or his family she should visit only once and recommend that the patient consulted the doctor. If the patient was not willing to do this she should not go again. This regulation which continued for many years after the health service came into being, determined the pattern of home nursing care for many years and accounts for the fact that general practitioners prescribed nursing care for patients, deciding which patients needed nursing, when they needed it, and the nature of the service to be given. It is true that the district nurse was generally trusted by the doctor to assess what nursing was needed and recommend any other services once she was called to the patient. However it was not until doctors and nurses worked together as *partners in care* that the concept of a nursing diagnosis and nursing care plans became a reality, although it is still not unusual to find instances of medically prescribed nursing treatment.

THE STATUTORY SERVICE

Section 25 of the National Health Service Act 1946[2] laid upon the major local authorities the duty to: 'make provision in their area, whether by making arrangements with voluntary organizations for the employment of nurses or by themselves employing nurses, for securing the attendance of nurses on persons who require nursing in their homes'. It is doubtful if the civil servants who framed the bill realized how many resources would be needed if the intention of the section was ever to be fully implemented.

The Act brought to all a more comprehensive service. Each person registered with a general practitioner and was entitled to consult him when necessary. Drugs, dressings and some nutrients could be prescribed for the patient. If the doctor thought he needed nursing he would ask the district nurse to call. The small charge for nursing care was discontinued. The work of the district nurses increased once they were freed from the constraint of assessing the patient's capacity to pay for care, and more people were entitled to their services, also certain new treatments became available for patients at home.

The first five years of the health service were years of optimism. The belief that disease diagnosed and treated early was controllable gave way only slowly to the realization that the child who escapes infectious disease lives on to suffer other traumas. It may be that the patient cured of tuberculosis develops diabetes in middle age. There was no awareness of how an increasingly elderly population was likely to strain the resources of the health service and be the major concern of all health workers in the eighties. In those years, the district nurses were sure of their place in the new system of health care. They accepted the thanks and praise of their patients, who for the most part found the help offered more personal and more compassionate than they had been led to expect. They saw no reason why given time general practitioners, hospital colleagues and health visitors should not recognize that they had special skills and accept them as partners in caring.

THE INQUIRIES OF THE FIFTIES AND SUBSEQUENT CHANGES

If the late forties were the years of anticipation, the fifties were years of soul searching. Working parties were set up by the government to look into the recruitment, field of work, and training of health visitors,[3] the training of district nurses,[4] and at the end of the decade into the employment and training of social workers.[5] A survey into the work of the general practitioner was also carried out by Taylor on behalf of the BMA.[6] Of all the reports that were published during that period the report into district nursing was the most limited, and it was a bitter disappointment to district nurses. Whereas the other reports called for more workers who were better prepared to cope with the increasing demands of their patients and clients, the report on the training of district nurses called for a reduction in the training period from six months to four. It was said, the improved standards of housing and improved education of the public made the task of the nurse less demanding than when she had worked in the abject poverty previously encountered in some patients' homes.

The profession was angry as well as disappointed, too late they realized that they had not been well represented; out of the seventeen members of the working party there were six nurses, only two of whom had any experience of district nursing. They were Miss Merry, General Superintendent of the Queen's Institute of District Nursing, and Miss

Treleavan, Senior Superintendent Ranyard District Nurses. Both ladies protested against the decision of the working party. Miss Merry and Dr Struthers, Medical Officer of Health for Holborn and Westminster, who was a member of the council of the Queen's Institute, wrote a minority report arguing the case for retaining the six months training. Two years after the report was published, Robin Turton, Minister of Health, addressed the annual meeting of the Queen's Institute and announced that the government was accepting the working party report and the training for district nursing would be reduced. The reduction was to be from six months to four, with a further reduction for certain nurses who had already spent eighteen months in district nursing, or who held certain post-certificate qualifications. He also said that any local authority wishing to establish their own training might do so, and that an advisory committee would be set up to help them.

This was done in 1957,[5] the committee had the following terms of reference: 'To advise the Minister on matters relating to the training and examination procedure for its national certificate in district nursing'. Its main object was to devise a four months training course and an examination system for registered nurses who wished to become district nurses.[7] A national certificate was to be awarded to all successful candidates. In 1959 the Panel of Assessors was established on the recommendation of the Advisory Committee to advise the Minister on schemes of training submitted by local authorities or the existing voluntary bodies for approval. The Panel was to become the validating body for district nurse training in the United Kingdom until it was superseded by the Council and National Boards set up under the Nurses, Midwives and Health Visitors Act 1979.[8]

Until 1967 the number of local authorities providing their own training was relatively small, the majority of students qualified through courses organized by the Queen's Institute of District Nursing. The Institute was a voluntary organization which for over seventy years had trained district nurses and coordinated the work of the many local voluntary nursing associations throughout the country. The Council of the Institute had anticipated being asked to serve as the advisory committee to the Minister and had suffered a very severe rebuff when the advisory committee recommended the establishment of the Panel of Assessors. The Queen's Institute was required to submit its scheme for approval. This it did reducing it in length to comply with the Panel's regulations and accepting the Advisory Committee's outline syllabus, until 1967. It then suddenly announced that it would cease awarding its certificate after the May examination in 1968.

This was the end of a tradition in which district nurses were trained for work where they were not supported by a network of social services, or extensive medical loan departments. It was said that the Queen's training homes superintendents prepared their students to improvise as though they were all going to work in some isolated outpost. This was an exaggeration but it was true that they maintained a high standard of work by training their staff to carry out certain standard and rather inflexible procedures.

This was necessary as some treatments brought hazards to staff as well as help for patients. The administration of streptomycin by injection to patients with tuberculosis for example led to the control of the disease and the closure of beds in tuberculosis hospitals. The numbers of visits paid by nurses to give these injections however ran into thousands and a long term effect of giving streptomycin injections was to cause dermatitis among the nurses. At that time syringes and needles were boiled before and after use, frequently a blunt needle was used to draw up the fluid from the phial and the sharp needle substituted just before the air was expelled and the injection given. Streptomycin was frequently spilled and some was sprayed into the room, particularly onto the nurse's hands and face. Various procedures were devised to protect both the giver and the receiver of the drug from getting the irritant fluid on their skin. In 1953 a teaching film was made demonstrating a relatively safe technique of administration thereby setting a pattern of work which was followed with very little modification until the introduction of disposable syringes.

In the first ten years of the health service the demand for nursing equipment so far outstripped supply that staff working in large cities and suburban areas had to be as inventive as those in the highlands and islands. They boiled their instruments before and after use, and baked dressings in biscuit tins, making do with jugs and cups for dressing bowls, cardboard boxes for footrests and bed cradles. These methods were still used in the 1960s and reflected the simplicity of the care given.

Just as the local authorities failed to anticipate the demands that were to be made on the service, neither the Queen's Institute nor the Advisory Committee were able to devise an educational programme that really met the challenge of the changing times. The new training patterns developed by the individual local authorities were to prepare nurses to work in their own areas. After 1968 therefore the three or four month courses became in-service training. The staff once in post demanded the equipment they had been taught to use. They took their requests directly to the medical officer of health who was responsible for both the training and the service. In consequence there was an improvement in most areas in the supply of such items as: commodes, hoists, incontinence pads, disposable equipment and pre-sterilized dressings.

In 1968 the intention of the original Act was extended by the Health Service and Public Health Act 1968.[9] In addition to providing nursing care in the patient's home, local authorities were required to secure 'the attendance of nurses on persons who require nursing elsewhere than in their own homes'. Meredith Davis[10] suggests that this extension of work leads to greater involvement of home nurses in diagnosis, investigations and in the treatment of illness. This came about through their work with the primary health care team, particularly in the treatment rooms attached to the practices. Work among the elderly was certainly increased as patients were discovered in boarding houses and residential hotels. Old people's homes also were catering for an increasingly infirm clientelle who needed skilled nursing as well as care.

THE DEVELOPMENT OF THE CONCEPT OF PRIMARY HEALTH CARE

From 1950 when a New Zealand general practitioner wrote a critical survey of British General Practice[11] the quality of medical diagnosis and treatment given to the patient at home had been called in question. However a general opinion persisted that the system was right even when countries as diverse as the USA, the USSR, Sweden, Denmark and Norway were reducing home care in their urban areas. As a result attempts were made to improve rather than to change the practice[12,13].

It was necessary to improve the premises from which doctors worked, to enable them to use the new medical technology that was available. This would have been no problem had the health centres envisaged in the National Health Service Act 1946 been available. They had been delayed for many reasons including shortage of building materials in the post-war years, and the reluctance of practitioners to use the few that were built. Doctors feared that if they moved into local authority premises they would lose their autonomy. They were determined to resist any move that might in the long term result in primary medical care becoming a salaried service in the same way as hospital medical care. Most practitioners therefore continued to work from their isolated and relatively under-equipped surgeries. Grants and allowances were made to help them improve their premises as well as to employ secretarial help and receptionists.

In the 1950s and 1960s the nursing staff employed by the local authorities were gradually being attached to groups of doctors in general medical practice, working from the same premises, serving the same patients, having access to each other's records. These schemes extended the consultations between doctors to include nurses and health visitors. When this communication was started it was very much concerned with the doctors giving their orders to the nurses directly, and the nurses reporting back to them, but it soon became wider. The nurses had already established the principle of post-basic training for domiciliary work and they were ready to contribute to the decision making and the formulation of care plans. The range of care quickly extended into prevention and health education.

Many general medical practitioners recognized their own need for education and training if they were to meet the growing demand for medical care outside hospital,[14] particularly in respect of those conditions which were principally emotional or psychological. This led to a consideration of primary medical care as a special subject in the medical curriculum. This term gave way in the 1970s to primary health care and both the medical and nursing professions focused their attention on how their multidisciplinary teams should be organized,[15] and what patterns of communication were most effective.

In 1971 Hawthorne[16] compiled an extended bibliography called *The Nurse Working with the General Practitioner* in which she listed and evaluated research into joint schemes of working. Gilmore,[17] et al.[18] had already started their research which was published in 1974 as the *Work of the Nursing Team in General Practice* in which they studied six teams in terms of their work loads and their internal structures. In 1973 Hicks, at the request of the DHSS, started a review of Primary Health Care published in 1976 as a book of that name.[19] His work ranged over the literature and the research studies that have been influential in developing the concept of shared care that is the ideal of every team. He was not uncritical of all he found and constantly urged all professional workers to think clearly about the system of primary health care needed for the future.

The success or failure of attachment schemes depended on the preparation made by the nursing officers before the placements were made, on the quality of interaction between the team members and on the trust each had on the other's professional skills and judgements. There are still teams where not everyone knows in sufficient detail what the others do. There are some teams where there is little if any exchange of ideas, opinions and suggestions for better working. In some teams skills are not properly used, highly trained workers are used for tasks that do not require their expertise, or complicated decisions are made by one person alone without consultation.

TEAMWORK IN PRIMARY CARE

Several models of teamwork have developed throughout the country. In some cases the team in primary care is led by the senior general practitioner who decides who does what. In most cases discussion is freer, the nurses, midwives and health visitors expecting some share in the responsibilities for the work, commensurate with the special skills they bring to the practice. In some teams, groups of professionals each with their own hierarchy work together in the larger health centres rather as doctors and nurses work together in hospital.

In the 1970s a few teams in peer groups have emerged in which the various professionals work together as equals. The introduction of social workers into attachment schemes has yet to be fully evaluated. It may be that their influence will change the pattern of the groups they join, or it may accelerate the development of groups of equals. What is needed in the 1980s is research into the effectiveness of primary health care, so that some unit of patient satisfaction or of improved health status in a community may be used to evaluate these various administrative structures. What can be said is that good team work brings as a bonus job satisfaction for all staff and there is some reason to believe that the quality of care provided is improved.

One of the problems of teamwork, particularly multidisciplinary teamwork, was and still is that of role definition and the proper identification of function. The independence of the nurse has been curtailed by attachment to a larger team delivering home care, comprising doctors, health visitors, social workers, school nurses, practice nurses and secretaries, but the responsibilities she carries have widened. Those responsible for the original legislation creating the National Health Service had envisaged a period of great activity while the backlog of disease was overcome followed by a great improvement in the nation's health. They thought as a consequence the cost would gradually lessen and fewer people would need to be employed by the health authorities. In the event, the costs escalated, particularly the cost of maintaining the hospital service. Even in the 1980s there are still unmet needs, particularly among the chronic sick and handicapped. Yet the numbers of people employed in the service has increased and become more specialized.

Some patients were investigated and treated as outpatients who would previously have been admitted. Those who went into hospital were discharged sooner. Often when they came home they still needed nursing supervision and health teaching. Some of the more complicated treatments required patients to adopt different patterns of diet, of exercise and of life style.

It was impossible for the district nurse to give the skilled nursing that was needed without becoming fully aware of the patient's medical background and total therapeutic programme. There was a need therefore for better cooperation between general practitioners, hospital and district nursing service.

The concept of teamwork suggests that when members of various health care disciplines are brought together this will result in a better quality of patient care. The fundamental error is in believing that bringing people together automatically creates a team. A team is a developing organization, the quality of its work being determined by the interaction of the members. Doctors, district nurses, health visitors and social workers working in isolation will identify the part that they individually play in patient care, however when they are brought together as a team each individual contribution has to be examined in relation to that of every other team member and the composite contribution measured against the needs of the particular practice caseload or patient group.

Inefficient written communication seems traditional in the health care disciplines, each having evolved its own recording methods. Old and inadequate patterns of communication that have outlived their usefulness die hard, but must be unlearned before new patterns can be evolved leading to better mutual understanding. Unless meaningful reports are combined into case histories, and patient care plans, the patients are denied the benefit of cumulative data collection. Some information may be confidential to a particular worker and not necessarily relevant to the making of a patient care plan. Generally patients will agree to sharing their private affairs with a small team providing that they know who it is that is involved, why they want the information and the way in which they will use it. The pattern of record keeping, the relevance of certain material, and data that contribute to the evaluation of treatment should be discussed regularly by each team, in order to facilitate joint working and a proper team approach to caring.

When a team is working together in harmony the roles within the team will change according to the personalities of the team members and the particular set of circumstances. In the same way leadership will change, it is not the prerogative of the doctor to be the leader although it may be convenient and best in many instances.

A cautionary note was sounded in a work study of district nursing staff in 1976. McIntosh and Richardson[20] found that nurses attached to group practices still adopted the subordinate role which characterizes the nurse/doctor relationship in hospital and they did not have the near equality of partnership which comprises real teamwork. These researchers assessed the contact between district nurses and doctors for the purpose of communicating ideas about patient care. They found this contact depended upon the facilities available to the nurse. Many nurses began their morning or afternoon sessions in the surgery at times that coincided with the doctor's consulting hours. Others had no accommodation at the surgery and had to see patients there when the doctor was out, they therefore had to come in and catch him before or after his surgery if they had reports to make or needed to discuss problems. Some teams evolved formal meetings with a chairman. Some enjoyed informal meetings at which the health visitor might also be present.

General practitioners still have a lot to learn about the work of district nurses and their contribution to the health and wellbeing of the sick and the elderly on the practice lists but while the nurses are reluctant to express their own views it perpetuates the misuse of nursing time and underuse of their skills.

The district nurse in the team has an important duty laid down in Statute — developed subsequently in many official reports — and made explicit in her contracts of service. She has a legal responsibility to care for her patients and an ethical code which is generally accepted throughout the profession. It is important that she knows what she should be doing, knows how to do it, and has the personal and professional integrity needed to maintain the quality of nursing care delivered to patients in all circumstances.

In many multidisciplinary groups it is not difficult to give of one's best, indeed colleagues' expectations are generally high and district nurses are constantly being stretched, but there are other situations. Misunderstandings, low morale, conflict between group members or pressure of work can mitigate against good nursing practice and standards may fall. When this happens the nurse must strive to maintain her own standards of work, and by persuasion try to influence her colleagues to discuss their problems and those of the group. Only thus can different priorities be reconciled without the delivery of care being adversely affected. If this fails the nurse is very much alone and must turn for professional help to the senior nursing managers.

District nurses have another responsibility in addition to that of team members. They have teams of their own to lead. In the original attachment schemes the nurses worked in relative isolation, but the extension of their role in 1968 added to their duties and extended the range of their work. They then saw the need for colleagues who had different and less extensive preparation to work with them. The teams they wanted were comprised of state enrolled nurses and auxiliaries who could undertake the routine care of patients. These teams came slowly even though it was recognized that unless she was so supported the state registered district nurse would be unable to develop her role fully in the primary health care team.

HOSPITAL LIAISON SCHEMES

From the mid-1960s schemes of coordination and cooperation between community and hospital staffs and between the various advisory members of the different professions involved in patient care were being developed. The new towns and overspill developments provided opportunities for services to be planned in an integrated fashion. Health centres were beginning to be built. Health visitors were probably the most widely used members of staff in liaison arrangements between the community and the hospital. District nurses were particularly concerned with early discharge of patients, and the aftercare of those who had been ill. Some experimental schemes included joint medical appointments and the joint use of premises. The general practitioners however still saw themselves not as integral members of the service but as users of the hospital service facilities for their patients.

An investigation carried out by Skeet in 1969[30] drew attention to the plight of the patient discharged from hospital without sufficient follow up. This together with the Queen's Institute's studies of cooperation between hospital and community care gave impetus to several projects aimed at bridging the gap. Patients having radiotherapy, patients having surgery, patients admitted with incontinence, stoma patients, stroke patients and others were followed up in various areas.

Many studies of children connected early hospital admissions with disturbance of behaviour, leading up to and including the period of adolescence and Douglas stated in 1975[31] 'thought should be given to how far home care can be safely substituted for hospital care for small children, especially for those already under strain'.

The care of children at home had interested district nurses since the

1950s when three experimental schemes were mounted in Rotherham, Birmingham and Paddington. The Court Report[33] published in 1978 caused a re-examination of the resources needed to integrate hospital and home care. Although the schemes varied according to the special circumstances, they all endeavoured to provide a service that was complementary to the service already given by the health visitor and district nurse.

THE GROWTH OF THE NIGHT NURSING SERVICE

In some areas the district nursing service was prevented from giving the best possible care because of insufficient or unsuitably deployed staff. In some areas there was no provision for night nursing and little accommodation in hospitals or other institutions for the periodic admission of the long-term sick. The effectiveness of nursing care in the home often depends upon the help and cooperation of the family. They carry a heavy burden and require help and support from staff who have the time and ability to give advice and guidance. Relatives of the very sick or the very demanding also need some rest during the 24 hours. In the case of cancer patients, night nursing on some nights of the week has been provided by trained nurses or auxiliaries, paid for by the Marie Curie Foundation, in order to give the relative some respite from the intensive caring. Some local authorities were able to provide night sitters to stay with patients who needed constant attention but not nursing care.

There are several types of nursing needed at night. Some patients need drugs administered in the late evening, this is most usually maintenance drugs or antibiotics given to people who are at work during the day but who do not have access to occupational health nursing. Patients suffering from terminal illness frequently need sedation at night. Some crippled patients need to be put to bed at night. Most of this work is carried out by an evening nursing service from 6 p.m. to 11 p.m.. During the remainder of the night some form of emergency service is now provided in most areas. The night nurses administer drugs, carry out treatments if necessary, deal with such crises as blocked catheters, and supervise the unqualified night sitters. When the 1972 syllabus made explicit the need for student district nurses to have experience of night duty it appeared that the Department of Health intended that night nursing should be an integral part of community care, and a more systematic provision has developed in many urban areas, nurses being employed from 11 p.m. to 8 a.m.

THE NURSING TEAM

Most of the work in patients' homes is carried out in the daytime. Indeed one of the problems of caseload management is that most patients want to be visited in the morning. Some patients have an obvious need for an early visit, if they are very ill, in pain, need help to the toilet or are incontinent. It is usual for the nurse to visit after she has given insulin to her diabetic patients. Conflicting with the demands of the priority patients for time in the mornings is the need for the nurse to spend some time in the surgery when the doctor is there. In order to organize the time to best advantage nurses must share their patients and a team rather than a single nurse will attend any particular group of patients. These teams may comprise several state registered nurses, about twice as many enrolled nurses and perhaps a nursing auxiliary working together.

THE CONCEPT OF SUPPORT

Many patients visited are alone in the house at least during the daytime. The elderly are particularly vulnerable to falls, to infection, and to cold. Although the majority want to retain their independence in the familiar surroundings of their own homes, many can only achieve this if they are given advice on general health, safety, nutrition, finances and sources of help. Also they need to have confidence that the support services will be made available at the proper time. In the last ten years health counselling has become an increasingly important part of the work of the district nursing team in order to keep these elderly patients active and usefully occupied all their lives.

The support services provided by the Social Services Department such as home helps, meals-on-wheels, are essential to the care of the sick, the handicapped and the frail. Equally important are physiotherapy, occupational therapy, chiropody and speech therapy. In all patient care emphasis must always be on rehabilitation, and the maintenance of independence. The increased numbers of professional workers has not always increased the amount of care each patient receives. It is necessary to use these workers sparingly to foster mutual understanding in order to avoid conflicting advice, and in some cases to enable one worker to reinforce the advice given by another. For example, the work of the speech therapist with a stroke patient can be enhanced by good cooperation with the district nurse who will help the patient and his family practise the new techniques of speech. It can be nullified if the nurse fails to understand the principles that the therapist is teaching, even though she may with the best intention be trying to help the patient in her own way.

RESEARCH INTO THE SERVICE

In the 1960s nursing became research minded and nurses started to investigate their own problems. One of the early appointments of a research officer was made by the Queen's Institute, and in that post Hockey carried out some detailed studies of the work of the registered[21] and the enrolled district nurses,[24] as well as the relationships between hospital and domiciliary services.[22][23] Her studies set the pattern of many studies that were to be carried out in a variety of areas in the 1970s. The attachment schemes had increased the travelling time nurses needed to visit their patients, the report writing, telephoning and conferring with other workers increased, until the district nurse might easily be spending more time travelling and managing her caseload than giving nursing care to patients.

More investigations and surveys followed the appointment of a director of nursing service in each local authority.[25] She had responsibility for all community nurses and her attention was focused on the relative professional, auxiliary and clerical staffing needs of each branch of the service. Another even more urgent need to have specific information about the role and function of different workers was occasioned by the imminent reorganization of the health service[26] and the integration of the hitherto separate community nursing services into the total group of professional nurses within the newly created area health authorities. In the community patients were being discharged earlier, investigated and treated as outpatients and delivered home by ambulance as people in need of nursing care. Into their homes came other nurses, with special skills, many acting in a consultant role, there were for example psychiatric nurses, stoma care nurses, and nurses with special knowledge of pain in terminal illness.

The concept of a nurse consultant had been discussed in all branches of nursing, but as district nurses were concerned with a wide range of patients their skills were essentially general, and a few only acquired special expertise. The majority of the new style consultant nurses were therefore hospital based, patient rather than family orientated. They were less familiar than the nurses in the primary care team with the particular life styles of the patients. They did not always understand the environmental factors that might exacerbate the disease or modify the effects of treatment. The need to work with the specialist visitors added impetus to another trend in the seventies, that of trying to specify the special skills of domiciliary nursing.

In this changing climate of the late 1970s the service-based research tended to give way to patient studies, and investigations into the efficacy of certain treatment plans.

CHANGES IN ATTITUDES TO TRAINING

Once the National Certificate in District Nurse Training was established and local authorities started developing their individual schemes of training, the outline curriculum was modified to suit local situations. The Panel of Assessors situated within the then Ministry of Health, and served by a Ministry Nursing Officer as professional adviser, was gaining in stature. It had sufficient standing in 1969 to oppose a suggestion made by the General Nursing Council that the community option might in some cases be a period of twelve weeks with the district nursing service and qualify the student upon registration for the National Certificate. There was a precedent, all the experimental integrated courses of nurse education include district nursing and health visitor training. In these special forms of nursing education the maximum use was made of the common core of knowledge required in the different fields of nursing and the placement of the students in the community with the district nurses was, as the title of the courses suggests, integrated into and extended by other experiences outside the hospital.

Not all district nurses approved of the integrated schemes, and certainly there was no support for the idea that similar placements could be extended to general nurse training. Even when it was suggested that following a twelve week placement the nurse upon qualification should work a further four weeks to bring the total time up to that required for the post-qualification student it aroused no enthusiasm. Backed by professional approval the Panel of Assessors insisted that no general approval could be given, for an integration of district nursing and general nurse training, and that any and every scheme must be submitted to them for scrutiny.

In 1970 the Committee on Nursing was set up under the chairmanship of Professor Asa Briggs to review the role of the nurse and midwife in hospital and in the community.[28] Among the Committee recommendations was that for a Central Council for the Training of Nurses, Midwives and Health Visitors in the United Kingdom with national boards for each country.

The recommendations were not formulated into an Act until 1979[29] and the implementation was delayed into the 1980s. While the original

report made suggestions about the pattern of the training programmes
the time lag between publication of the report and implementation of the
legislation made many detailed proposals out of date before the newly
created statutory body was ready to undertake any curriculum development.

District Nurse training meanwhile had not stood still. In 1971 a
National Certificate in District Nursing was issued to state enrolled
nurses who had followed a ten week course. Practical work instructors
who undertook the practical teaching of the registered students were
involved after 1969 in the assessment procedure for their students. After
1974 experienced district nurses were required to undertake a special
teaching course of at least fifteen days before practising as practical work
instructors.

In 1973, with regard to the increasing amount of teaching undertaken
by district nurse tutors, with registered and enrolled students for the
Certificate, to student nurses on the Community Option, and during
inservice training programmes for community staff, a year's formal training in teaching was required by any district nurse who wished to be a
tutor. Also every course in district nursing submitted to the Panel for
approval had to be organized by a qualified tutor.

In 1976 the Panel of Assessors set up a working party to devise an
improved syllabus based on the existing district nursing syllabus without
prejudice to the implementation of the Briggs (Committee of Nursing)
recommendations. The working party reported within the year,[30]
recommending a much more comprehensive course of education lasting
six months followed by three months supervised practice. It integrated
into the teaching insights from psychology, sociology, epidemiology and
social policy. The working party believed that such a demanding course
as they wished to see established would need to have special entry
requirements and they suggested five subjects at ordinary level in the
General Certificate of Education. The syllabus was warmly received by
the profession who recognized the need for education to meet the changing demands of the job.

District nurses meanwhile were not sure that the proposed legislation
to set up the new Central Council for Nursing, Midwifery and Health
Visiting would safeguard their interests. In 1977–78 they organized
themselves into a protest movement, arranging meetings, sending peti-
tions to the Secretary of State for the Social Services and the Ministers of
Health demanding a standing committee to advise the Central Council on
all district nursing matters. There was also a general call for training to be

mandatory, and practice as a district nurse was forbidden to anyone who did not hold the national certificate. There was no immediate response to this protest but in the following year the Panel of Assessors was reconstituted, its membership was increased from eleven to twenty and one month later in October 1978 the Health Ministers announced that a new curriculum based on the recommendations of the working party, but lasting only six months, was to be introduced in Autumn 1981 and that training should be mandatory for employment as a district nurse. In March 1980 a further working party report was issued, this time on the Education and Training of the State Enrolled Nurse.[31]

THE EXTENDED ROLE OF THE DISTRICT NURSE

The role of the nurse is continually developing and nurses are constantly acquiring new skills to meet new needs, but new skills require new knowledge which implies further training, and before nurses undertake new work they must be aware of the legal implications that follow. In 1974 a joint working party was set up representing the Association of Nurse Administrators, the Health Visitors Association, the Royal College of Nursing and the British Medical Association. Their findings were incorporated in a health circular in 1977,[32] in which they saw two ways in which the role of the nurse was extended in addition to the continuous process mentioned above; one when the doctor delegates a specific task and another when the nurse must respond to an emergency. In delegation the doctor remains responsible for the patient but the nurse is responsible for carrying out the delegated tasks competently. In an action for damages a nurse may be held legally liable if it can be shown either that she has failed to exercise the skills properly expected of her, or that she has undertaken tasks she was not competent to perform. The doctor may be held to be guilty of negligent delegation if it can be shown that he conferred authority on a nurse to perform a task which was either outside the scope of the duties she was normally expected to perform, or for which she had no special qualification.

Health Authorities were asked to review areas where delegation to nurses was desirable. The following procedures were included in most authorities' lists of treatments that might be considered an extension of the nurse's normal duties:

1. Venepuncture
2. Suturing superficial wounds
3. Administration of intravenous drugs
4. Emergency endotracheal intubation

5. Changing tracheostomy tubes
6. Defibrillation
7. Removal of foreign bodies from the ear
8. Vaccination and immunization

It is not necessarily new for nurses to carry out some of these procedures, many do so very competently but their skills are not always based on knowledge but taught as a technique only, based on trial and error. Knowledge is an essential part of the skill if nursing practice is to be a professional activity. It is necessary for nurses to be sure that they do have enough knowledge to perform any procedures safely. Where teaching is not included in basic or post-basic training, or where training was not enough to ensure thorough knowledge this should be reported to the Nursing Officer and help sought in gaining the theoretical base and supervised practice until competence is assured.

There is an extension to the role of the district nurse which is not strictly clinical. While people are expecting more and more from the health service seeking help for minor conditions that earlier generations would have treated themselves or just tolerated, not all levels of the population are getting equal care. District nurses as well as other members of the primary care team must develop health care in areas of multiple deprivation. Many district nurses are aware of the potential help health supervision can bring to the elderly and are asking for clinics to monitor the hearing, sight, mobility, respiratory competence and blood pressure of their patients, initiating treatment promptly and giving health education when it is most likely to be received and used.

Miniaturizing of equipment will enable more treatment to be carried to the surgeries and to patients' homes. Monitoring vital signs, investigations and treatments formerly carried out only in specialized units and hospitals may soon be available to the primary health care team and district nurses will be in the forefront of these developments.

CONCEPTS AND PRINCIPLES

These concepts and principles range from the very simple shorthand that is used to describe care given, to the more complex influences that have given direction to the consideration of a theoretical basis to the practice of district nursing. The ideas are simple, but sometimes difficult to apply.

COMPREHENSIVE PATIENT CARE

Because district nursing was originally ordered by doctors it was frequently associated with the giving of prescribed treatments. Nurses quickly recognized that they could often contribute to the patient's recovery and comfort by giving more care than was ordered. Several different terms were used as a shorthand to represent approaches to patient care.

General nursing care was the term used to describe the basic physical care such as bathing, care of the skin, positioning the patient, attending to his oral hygiene and pressure areas. It also included such teaching as was needed to enable the patient's family to care for him between visits.

As the profession became aware of the emotional, social and behavioural implications of disease they needed a term to represent the enlarged perspective so that the assessment made would automatically include these factors. So the term *comprehensive care* was coined. A further extension covering the aforementioned and including the contribution that might be made by other community services such as meals-on-wheels and home helps was in the 1960s called by the term *total patient care*.

The concept of the nursing process has now incorporated the process of assessment for total patient care. This is preferable because the concept includes not only assessment, but also planning and giving care, and the evaluation of the care given. It implies an individual plan made for the patient rather than a blanket form of care, but most important it is a term that is common to all nursing both within the hospital and the community, that will further an exchange of nursing knowledge within an increasingly integrated profession.

CONTINUITY OF CARE

Illness is only an episode in the life of a patient, but within many illnesses there is need for care in different situations. The patient who is admitted to hospital from the community or who attends the outpatient department for a consultation should take information of their treatment and the results observed by the primary care team to aid diagnosis and facilitate the choice of further treatment. Likewise the team in the community needs adequate briefing if they are to receive a patient home from hospital to continue care uninterrupted.

Patients have frequently been their own message carriers between hospital and the community. This is often quite satisfactory but not entirely reliable, and it is the most ill and the most anxious patients who are likely to mishear or misunderstand instructions given to them in hospital. To put the patient further into the picture and involve him and his family in the decision making about his treatment is a relatively new idea. This consultation process enables the more articulate patient to question the consultant and others, but the more anxious do not always enjoy the process. It involves the medical and nursing team in much heart searching and anxiety when the patient refuses the treatment that is recommended and they have to stand by him despite this.

Quality of care depends upon trust existing between the team and the patient. Where the patient is visited less frequently and he or his family increasingly take on the caring role, continuity of care becomes very important. This may not be nursing care by one person only but visiting by a group who know each other, use the same approach, give the same advice and the same encouragement. This does not happen by chance but only if care is taken over the interpretation of the nursing plan and communications between the group members are clear, concise and accurate.

THE CONTAINMENT OF DISEASE

This is the organization of work in such a manner as to prevent disease spreading and where possible ensuring that the adverse effect upon others is minimal.

Disease within the patient may be contained by the prevention of complication. Thus the patient with paralysis nursed in a position where he is able to have each joint put through the range of movement to prevent contractures, is going to be in a better position to work towards mobility as soon as this is practical.

When tuberculosis was one of the more common diagnoses found in the district nurse's caseload, it was necessary to be careful not to risk contracting the disease or carrying it to other patients. However, infectious disease is not the only condition that had implications for the well-being of those caring for the patient. The heavy patient can cause back injury to nurse and relatives if care is not taken to learn and practise the proper way to lift. Nursing a patient through an exhausting terminal illness can produce severe stress symptoms in relatives. While sorrow and grief are not entirely relieved by nursing or social support, however sensitively given, the amount of distress and the subsequent pain of bereavement can be lessened by careful support and counselling.

Referral of patients to other workers is frequently necessary and skilful referral is essential if the effects of illness are to be reduced and the best care is to be provided. The use of other workers' expertize depends upon an attitude of mind that seeks widely for the most appropriate help for patients, an absence of possessiveness and a capacity to share information. It is necessary to be able to communicate essential knowledge about the needs of the patient without revealing confidences that have been given in the course of treatment, in times of stress, or when the patient was feeling particularly dependent. Referrals have to be accepted before the referrer can relinquish her responsibility for the situation.

Leaving a message for a doctor does not necessarily constitute a referral and there is no reduction in the nurse's responsibility until he has actually intervened himself. Referrals to social workers may not necessarily mean that a visit will be paid immediately and if delay occurs the patient must be able to rely upon the nurse in the meantime.

Referral within an integrated team should be a simple matter as each team member should know what their colleagues can do in a given set of circumstances, how they approach their work, what information they need and how easy or difficult it is at any particular time to accept new patients. Referrals outside the immediate team are frequently made by telephone or by letter. Written communications and written confirmation of telephone messages are preferable when detailed material has to be passed between colleagues who are not in very close contact. It may be that the well-written nursing process which includes contributions from all care-givers will be the best instrument the service has for accurate referral and the prevention of error and the containment of disease.

REFERENCES

1. STOCKS, M. (1958). *A Hundred Years of District Nursing*. London: Allen & Unwin.
2. *The National Health Service Act*, 1946, London: HMSO.
3. *An Inquiry into Health Visiting*: Report of a Working Party on the Field of Work, Training and Recruitment of Health Visitors (1956). London: Ministry of Health.
4. MINISTRY OF HEALTH, (1955). *Report of the Working Party on the Training of District Nurses*. London: HMSO.
5. *Report of the Working Party on Social Workers in the Local Authority Health and Welfare Services*. (1959). London: HMSO.
6. TAYLOR, S. (1954). *Good General Practice*. Oxford: Oxford University Press.
7. *The Training of District Nurses*. (1959). Report of the Advisory Committee. London: HMSO.
8. *The Nurses, Midwives and Health Visitors Act, 1979*. London: HMSO.
9. *The Health Services and Public Health Act, 1968*. London: HMSO.
10. MEREDITH DAVIES, J.B. (1979). *Community Health, Preventive Medicine and Social Services*, 4th Ed. London: Baillière Tindall.
11. COLLING, J. 'A Survey of British General Practice', *Lancet*, 25th March, 1950.

12. *Report of the Committee on General Practice within the NHS*. (1954). London: HMSO.
13. TAYLOR, S. (1954). *Good General Practice*. Oxford: Oxford University Press.
14. *The Field of Work of the General Practitioner*: Report of the Subcommittee of the Standing Medical Advisory Committee (1971). London: HMSO.
15. *The Organisation of Group Practice*: a Report of a Subcommittee of the Standing Medical Advisory Committee, (1971). London: HMSO.
16. HAWTHORNE, P.J. (1971). *The Nurse Working with the General Practitioner:* An evaluation of research and a review of some of the literature. London: DHSS.
17. GILMORE, M. (1970). 'A Pilot Study of the Work of the Team in General Practice'), *The Medical Officer*, 124.
18. GILMORE, M., BRUCE, N. & HUNT, M. (1974). *The Work of the Nursing Team in General Practice*, Council for the Education and Training of Health Visitors. London: HMSO.
19. HICKS, D. *Primary Health Care*: A Review – DHSS (1976). London: HMSO.
20. McINTOSH, J.B. & RICHARDSON, I.M. (1976). *Work Study of District Nursing Staff*, Scottish Health Service Studies No. 37, Scottish Home and Health Dept.
21. HOCKEY, L. (1966). *Feeling the Pulse*: A Study of District Nursing in Six Areas, London: Queen's Institute of District Nursing.
22. HOCKEY, L. (1968). *Care in the Balance*: A Study of Collaboration between Hospital and Community. London: Queen's Institute of District Nursing.
23. HOCKEY, L. & BUTTIMORE, A.A. (1970). *Cooperation in Patient Care*. London: Queen's Institute of District Nursing.
24. HOCKEY, L. (1972). *Use or Abuse*? A Study of the Work of the State Enrolled Nurse in the Local Authority Nursing Service. London: Queen's Institute of District Nursing.
25. *The Report of the Working Party on Management Structure in the Local Authority Nursing Service*. (1969). London: DHSS.
26. *The National Health Service Reorganisation Act, 1973*.
27. *The Report of the Committee on Nursing* (Chairman, Prof. Asa Briggs). (1972). London: DHSS (Cmnd 5115) HMSO.
28. *The Report of the Working Party on the Education and Training of District Nurses* (SRN/RGN), The Panel of Assessors for District Nurse Training (UK). (1976). London: DHSS.
29. *Report of the Working Party on the Education and training in District Nursing for the State Enrolled Nurse*, Panel of Assessors for District Nurse Training (UK). (1980). London: DHSS.
30. SKEET, M. (1967). *Home from Hospital*: A Survey of Patients Discharged from Hospital, Dan Mason Research Committee.
31. DOUGLAS, J.W.B., Early Hospital Admissions and Later Disturbances of Behavior and Learning, *Developmental Medicine and Child Neurology*, 456–480.
32. Health Circular, *The Extending Role of the Clinical Nurse*, Legal Implications and Training Requirements, HC(77)22, (June 1977). London: DHSS.
33. *Fit for the Future* (The Court Report). The Report of the Committee on Child Health Services (1976) DHSS. London: HMSO.

SECTION ONE

The Professional Skills

CHAPTER 2

The Nursing Process

The Nursing Process is a method of nursing management whereby the unique needs of the patient and his family may be identified. The nursing care plan which is jointly agreed by the nurse and the patient enables the nurse to review care, and for nursing colleagues to know more precisely what is expected at any visit. The increasing sophistication of the service places an obligation of accountability on each professional person. Responsibility for her own performance is stressed in the latest curriculum for Registered District Nurses,[1] as the success of cure or comfort depends upon the contribution of many professionals in the present health service. In fulfilling this obligation of identifying nursing needs, essential areas of cooperation with doctors and other health and social workers are clarified.

It is a new approach to 'total' or 'comprehensive patient care'. These earlier terms, which were used by all nurses, had a particular meaning for district nurses who of necessity have had to consider the patient in the setting of his own home and family. The two most important changes implicit in the nursing process are the detailed consideration of the patient as a person and the preparation of a nursing care plan. In the past, nursing documentation has tended to record only nursing intervention[2]. Using the nursing process, nursing records formulate a plan of care based on a nursing assessment which is followed by identification of nursing objectives, nursing intervention and continuous evaluation of care.

Many district nurses are now familiar with the nursing process model of four or five phases (Fig. 1). While this model is of obvious value when devising a system of care for the individual patient, it is also applicable to the district nurse's total workload. In a WHO Report on Community Nursing in 1974,[3] the Committee described the role of community health

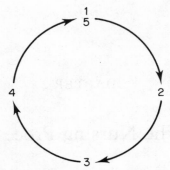

Fig. 1. The nursing process model.

1. *Assessment*. History and observations
   Identification of patients
   'problems' or 'nursing needs'

2. *Goals or Objectives*. Long term
   Short term

3. *Plan of nursing care*.
   Actions by whom, when and how.

4. *Progress*. Monitoring progress
   Evaluating progress
   Reviewing progress

5. *Re-assessment*.

workers in conjunction with the patient, family and community representatives. There the nursing process included:

1. Assessment of 'community health states'.
2. Identification of problems and the development of service priorities and plans.
3. Implementation of the 'agreed upon services'.
4. Evaluation and the determination 'of measures to be used to reflect attainment of objectives and of safety and quality of care.'

The principle of consultation and consideration of the recipient is similar whether the community is participating in preparing objectives for health care, and when the patient is involved in planning his own care.

A radical change of attitude may be required by the nursing profession if this principle is to be wholly accepted.

Many books and articles have now been written by authors in the United Kingdom featuring 'the nursing process' or 'the process of nursing' as one group of writers preferred it to be called.[4]

Professionalism has been defined in various ways but most definitions include the possession of a specialized body of knowledge acquired by a specific educational programme. The professional person bases her practice on knowledge and research; follows certain principles and ideals; is critical of her own performance and is service orientated. Nursing must therefore embody an underlying process or pattern.[5]

The professional education of the nurse is given an added dimension during district nurse education.

The district nurse meets a wide variety of patients who may be with, or without families or friends. Each patient has different physical, emotional and social resources. It is impossible to choose a typical patient but it may be useful to illustrate the application of the nursing process to one patient before moving on to consider more general issues raised by its practice. The format or structure may be modified, but the basic precepts described earlier are the essentials to be grasped.

In this example the patient was referred to the district nurse by the general medical practitioner at the time of a family crisis precipitated by the death of the patient's wife. The elderly wife had looked after her severely handicapped husband, and apart from the visits of the family doctor, the wife and husband had supported each other, declining offers of outside help. At the time of the initial contact the nurse was conscious that the household had undergone a dramatic change, and was very different from that household a week earlier. The information recorded on the history sheet was collated from the patient's responses, the daughter's remarks and the nurse's own observations (Table 1).

IDENTIFICATION OF PROBLEMS

Those activities which the patient was unable to attend to himself became apparent during the first few visits and thus his nursing needs or problems were identified. 'Nursing problems arise when people are unable to meet certain health related needs.'[6] This patient's inability to voice his needs completely may be the result of shock following his wife's death, or it may be that the patient had previously been inarticulate and resisted any movement. The immediate problems as observed must be simply stated. Although the nurse needed to seek further information from the general practitioner, her own professional expertise would guide her when assessing the extent to which the mental confusion and limb spasticity were recent changes due to the bereavement, or other causes.

Table 1. Example of Nursing History Sheet incorporated into Patient Record System

Surname	Forename	Sex	Marital state	Date of birth	Date of 1st visit
BROWN	Albert	M	Widower	6.12.1900	1.11.1980

Full address	Tel: No:	Occupation	Religion
Ground Floor Flat,		Retired railway guard	
6, High Street,	New Town		
	Access	Special instructions	
	Front door	Daughter at home temporarily	

Next of kin.	Name and Relationship	Full address	Tel: No:
Daughter	Mrs Ann SMITH	First Floor Flat,	At work 333/444
S/A as patient		6, High Street,	
		New Town	

General Practitioner	Tel: No:	Referred by (Name and address)
Dr C.	777-666	Dr C.

Diagnosis(es) to District Nurse	Reason for referral	Hospital attendance
Arteriosclerosis	Series of mild strokes	None at present
		Ward/Outpatient Department

Composition of household   *Patients dependants*
Daughter, son-in-law. 2 grandchildren
(12 and 14 yrs) in upstairs flat

Housing (tick)   Owner – Local Authority   Rented
                                                                                  √

Bungalow	Semi	Detached	Flat	Other
	√		Groundfloor	

Financial state (not essential)

Retirement pension

NURSING ASSESSMENT

History of Present Condition

Wife died two days ago.
Hypertension.
Series of mild strokes, dates not known.
Was getting up, and sitting in chair each day with help from wife.

Previous Health:

Daughter says he has been confined to the house for the past two years.

General Appearance (Colour/posture) :

Pale thin man – very tall. Stiffness of arms and legs, particularly when lying in bed.

Ability to communicate/response to questions:

Tries to enter into conversation when spoken to directly, sometimes responds inappropriately, breaks off and becomes tearful.
Feeling expressed: Cries easily, fluctuates between tears and humour.
Speech: Repeats well known jokes. Difficulty in remembering recent events and is frustrated by this.
Mobility: Can take a few steps when supported on both sides. Some spasticity and lack of co-ordination in movement. Unable to lift himself from a lying position to sitting position.
Vision: Difficult to assess, cannot concentrate to read. Does not wear his glasses.
Hearing: Sometimes remarks have to be repeated.

Mouth and Teeth:

Tongue coated.
Dentures

Nutrition (Usual eating/drinking habits and preferences) :

Usually eats ordinary meals but has a very small appetite.
(Wife previously prepared meals)

Daughter offers him extra teas and coffee, but he rarely drinks all of them.
Used to enjoy a glass of beer in the evenings when neighbour visited.

Pain:

Leg movements painful, particularly after lying in bed.

Social Activities:

Neighbours call in frequently
Watches TV
Used to be very interested in music—played in local brass band.

Sleep Pattern:

Wakes during night but does not call for attention. Daughter hears him talking to himself.
Sleeps in chair during day.

Condition of Skin:

Needs help with washing and shaving.
Elbows red.
Groins sore—from urinary incontinence.

Urinary Function:

Frequency and some lack of control.
Bed wet in morning. Unable to answer questions about this.
Daughter suspects this may be long standing problem.

Bowel Function:

None during last two days.
Senekot tabs on table.

OBSERVATIONS AT 1st ASSESSMENT MADE BY NURSE

Temperature:	37	*Height: (Approximately)*
Pulse:	60	6ft. 4 ins
Respiration:	18	
(Expectoration)		*Weight: (Approximately)*

Blood Pressure: 180   Thin, has lost weight gradually.
                           100   Used to weigh 15 stones.

Urinalysis: No albumen or sugar
             Heavy deposit
             Strong smell of ammonia

Further relevant information

DRUGS CURRENTLY IN USE, DOSE AND FREQUENCY

1 Hydrochlorothiazide
  100 mg each morning
2 Nitrazepam – 5 mg at night

Any known allergic reaction:

Hospital treatments:

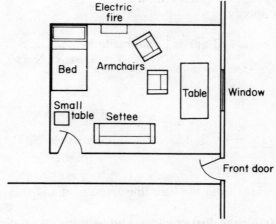

Fig. 2. Arrangement of the patient's room.

FACILITIES

Sick Room:

    Front room lounge.
    Bed in corner, near fire, very little space.

Bathroom, washing and toilet facilities:

  Bathroom downstairs off kitchen.
  Hot water from gas heater in kitchen.

Accessibility of rooms to patient:

  Patient has not been out of room recently.

Heating arrangements:

SUPPORTING SERVICES IN USE AT 1st VISIT

Health Visitor	—
Social Worker	—
Home Help	—
Meals-on-Wheels	—
Laundry Service	—
Chiropody	—
Social Security	not known
Other (please specify)	—

First assessment, and nursing plan made by:...........................
                                              District Nurse

THE GOALS OF CARE

These are decided from the base line assessment and they dictate the action plan.

  In this example the district nurse is brought into a complex situation where practical help is required at a time of emotional crisis. The philosophy of the nursing process is that the patients viewpoint is considered first and the problems looked at through his eyes. While this does not mean that the nurse necessarily complies with all the patient's requests, it does prevent the nurse from making decisions without fully considering his feelings or explaining her actions. A nurse could not be insensitive to the patient's feelings of grief initially, but this could quickly

Table 2 (A) Nursing Care Plan

Date	Problem	Goal	Action	By whom	Review
1.11.80	Grief (wife died two days ago)	To receive support during initial days of mourning	Comfort patient Allow time for patient to talk if he wishes	SRN and SEN	
1.11.80	Communication (due to illness, shock or slight deafness)	To overcome speech difficulties	Talk directly to patient Speak slowly Give short instructions Observe hearing and check with doctor	SRN teaches other care givers	1 week
1.11.80	Mouth dry Tongue 'furred'	To prevent discomfort and oral infection	Mouth washes morning and evening Dentures to soak overnight Jug of water to be placed near patient and daughter to give half a glass of water each time she enters room	SRN SEN Daughter	Daily
1.11.80	Unable to care for personal hygiene or undress himself due to lack of coordination of movement and spasticity of limbs	To promote skin healing, and prevent deterioration of skin condition	Morning bath and inspection of pressure areas. Help to dress Evening visit to wash and change clothes. Encourage patient to assist with washing and dressing.	SRN and SEN	1 week

Table 2 (B) Nursing Care Plan

Date	Problem	Goal	Action	By whom	Review
1.11.80	Unable to move safely from bed to chair due to lack of space	Adequate space and safety to practice walking	Discuss with daughter removal of the settee, the provision of a fireguard and the placing of commode near the bed	Son-in-law	2.11.80
1.11.80	Inadequate intake of food due to complete change of routine	To recover previous appetite	Small savoury meals as specimen diet sheet (patient dislikes sweet dishes) Water and fruit drinks throughout the day (Diuretic tablet after breakfast) Continue evening glass of beer	Daughter	Daily
1.11.80	Wakeful during night	Promote sleep	Nitrazepam, 5mg at 9 pm Observe sleep pattern	Daughter	3.11.80
1.11.80	Concerned about dependency on daughter, and what will happen when she returns to work	To devise a plan for future care. Listen to anxieties expressed	Ask General Practitioner history and discuss the advisability of full medical and social assessment within a week Consult occupational therapist about temporary	SRN	As events progress

funeral in three days time

Date	Problem	Aim	Nursing action	Nurse	Evaluation
1.11.80	Incontinence of urine at night and occasionally in day	To ascertain causes of incontinence, and lessen the effects	Check frequency and quantity of urinary output, and save specimen for laboratory test	SRN	Urine report
			Consult GP about incontinence, and special cream for sore groins		
	Unable to position urinal in bed		Apply waterproof cream to buttocks and hips		Daily
			Sit patient on commode after morning bath		
			Teach patient and relative how to position urinal		
			Consult District Charge Nurse regarding appropriate appliance		in 1 week
1.11.80	Spasticity of limbs	To promote maximum mobility	Help patient from bed to commode, to armchair by supporting each side	SRN and SEN or one nurse with help of daughter or neighbour	Daily
		To prevent increasing spasticity as a result of immobility	Gentle passive movements to lower limbs before getting up		
			Encouraging active purposeful movements when washing and dressing		

fade from the picture unless grief was recorded as a problem and given consideration in the nursing care plan. Similarly unless the various phsyical problems regarding immobility, loss of bladder control, spasticity of limbs, etc., were each detailed, the nurse could sum up the situation by stating that the patient needs 'general nursing, with special attention to pressure areas'. Where more explicit directives are not left, the patient will receive as little or as much attention as each subsequent nurse deems temporarily necessary. The contribution by those in attendance between the nurse's visits might not be fully acknowledged or at best covered in conversations by the nurse and relative. Any new nurse visiting would be dependent upon a written message, or a verbal message possibly by telephone, which may not go further than the task to be performed. The nursing plan in the house ensures quality and continuity of nursing attention.

The nurse who is studying the patient will be much more attentive to details such as his response to conversations, the content of his diet, and his reaction to medication because these have been written into the nursing plan. It may be necessary to ask if the furniture can be arranged to enable the patient to have a clear space to move when being helped from bed to chair. A table may be required by the bedside so that the patient can reach for a drink at night, or be given a more comfortable bed bath. While the nurse's own health and safety have to be remembered, that which is ultimately most effective in nursing care would not run counter to this. The nurse can get help from other disciplines such as the Occupational Therapist and from the family. Overcoming difficulties in delivering nursing care are part of the plan of action, these are the nurse's and not always patients' nursing problems.

In the example given, the district nurse's prime responsibility would be to her patient, the elderly widower; but in caring for him she also has an interest in the whole family and would see her role as offering solace and help to the daughter and her family. The nurse recognizes that the daughter's feelings of grief must be appreciated if immediate nursing plans are to be realistic. While recognizing that the daughter's grief may be affecting her receptiveness to teaching about the father's care the nurse may also make a major contribution to the daughter's subsequent health. In district nursing there is such a close relationship between the district nurse and the relatives that there may be occasions when the district nurse has to decide whether another member of the family is also another patient or client in need of help. It is probable that unless the daughter has a physical illness, any untoward long term psycho-social help for her may be obtained after discussion with other members of the primary health care team. The decision regarding the most suitable person to follow up the daughter's need for help would depend upon her particular area of need, and each team member's prime responsibility Their personal abilities and aptitudes may also determine who should help different members of the family, and whether one team member should act as key worker for the whole family.[7]

The continued contact of the district nurse with this family places her in a favourable position to become the key worker, but the nature of the problems, or availability of time may cause her to enlist help from other sources. The resources within the family may be sufficient without outside help. Whatever the circumstances the written care plan enables the nurse to monitor and evaluate progress. In this household it is unlikely that she would have more than one patient, but in others particularly where there are two elderly people she may have two patients. If this should happen she will have to decide whether two nursing care plans or a joint one will be most helpful to the patients.

THE NURSING HISTORY AND FRAMEWORK FOR ASSESSMENT

Different frameworks have been described to ensure that a full nursing history is obtained. The district nurse may decide that she can get to know her patients best by using one particular framework, or she may decide that by using a combination of different approaches she is prompted to think more widely. One approach may be more appropriate than another according to the context of the patient, e.g. 'the head to toe' approach may be the choice if the patient is alone and does not find it easy to communicate. Frameworks like computers are only as good as their users, and it is the thinking behind their use which decides their true value. Taking a nursing history is never a series of predetermined questions. It is an exploration of categories of needs and feelings which are common to everyone, but have particular significance according to the illness of the person whose nursing needs are being assessed. Whatever information the patient discloses pertaining to his health needs, it is reasonable for him to expect to know what action may be taken. He will also expect to be able to add to or change this information later.

The familiar compartments — physical, mental and socio-economic are useful starting points. When these are looked at in more detail it will be seen that there is considerable overlap between these categories, for example data which is primarily physical may impinge on mental and social activities. Lack of mobility due to a scalded foot will affect the mother's physical feelings and activities and her emotional state and therefore her ability to fulfill her social function as a housewife. The nurse has to decide whether 'frustration in not fulfilling her maternal role' is sufficiently great to warrant recording and therefore questions the need for subsequent nursing action.

Some nurses may prefer to use the life history approach when compiling a nursing history. The interviewer beginning by saying 'Tell me about yourself, were you born in this town?' and so on. The areas explored would be parents, siblings, position in family, health at school, and at work, marriage and subsequent family, leading to the present day and current illness. The current illness or dominating symptom is of obvious importance. The nurse needs to know the person's knowledge of his illness and diagnosis, and how he feels about any symptoms and treatment. The usual pattern of his life and whether this has been affected is also pertinent to the person's subsequent care. The activities of daily living, eating, sleeping, bowel and bladder action, the maintenance of warmth, comfort, and ability to care for personal hygiene all need to be considered. Occupation, leisure and family responsibilities also affect the persons nursing prospects and should be considered. Direct observation by the district nurse will often dispense with the need for questions.

THE HEAD-TO-TOE AND BODY SYSTEMS APPROACH

This has been recommended by some writers on the nursing process. A comprehensive picture of the patient can be built up from questions and observations beginning with the head, the facial expressions, complexion, hair, eyes, teeth, etc., working systematically downwards. This method can be seen to have similarities to the medical model of history taking, although the nurse would be relying on overt observations and answers to questions and not detailed clinical examinations. The nurse has the advantage in that the patient expects to undress for many aspects of nursing care. She may wish to make notes under the various body systems.

Mental State

Questions and observations under this heading might include such items as communications, memory, and the opportunities available for mental stimulation.

Special Senses

These are useful references for the nurse to keep in mind when checking the capabilities of the patient at home. Minor defects affect not only physical independence but social interaction, particularly in those patients suffering from multiple disabilities.

The Skin and Locomotor System

Questions on mobility and the ability to perform the various movements required in self care would be prompted by this heading, in addition to possible concentration on any affected limbs or joints. The nurse would also be reminded to look for any obstacles in the environment which might limit maximum mobility in the house.

Gastro-intestinal and urinary systems

Linked with this system would be enquiries about nutrition and possibly oral medication, bowel and micturition habits. Associated pain or discomfort might also be queried.

Respiratory System

Nasal catarrh, sore throat, breathlessness, expectoration, coughs might be uncovered when thinking of this heading.

Circulatory System

Direct observation by the nurse of colour, pulse, blood pressure, etc., would be appropriate under this heading as under any of those previously mentioned. Patients medications and the reactions would be relevant under any heading.

There may be other body systems which the nurse feels it would be valuable to include, if only to direct her thoughts to their possible significance. Perhaps the Reproductive System or Endocrine System would be useful prompters. In any event the nurse will probably decide to settle for some additional headings because everything does not fit into the systems categories. For example:

1. Verbal communications voice, speech, articulateness, ability to express his feelings
2. Relationships within the household
3. Reaction to illness
4. Ability to bath, cook, and care for himself within the limited facilities of the home
5. Socio-economic state

FUNDAMENTAL HUMAN NEEDS

The relationship of fundamental human need to the components of nursing as identified by Virginia Henderson[8] continues to be an excellent reference for all nurses. The list of fourteen basic human needs can be applied to any patient, and referred to when the nurse is assessing a patient's nursing needs. The adult patient transferred home early after abdominal surgery may experience difficulty with 'sleep and rest', so may the young child after a similar experience. The ordinary needs taken for granted in health, become prominent according to the illness. Henderson also points out that these are affected by age, temperament, social or cultural status, and the physical and intellectual capacity of the person.

A.H. Maslow[9] also identified basic needs beginning with those fundamental to survival and progressing to the satisfaction of the person's highest potential. Needs were placed in order of priority, and satisfaction of one group of needs led to concentration on the next group of needs. First physiological needs required fulfilment, i.e. breathing, nutrition, and those needs essential for physical survival. The next group were classed as safety needs; not only physical safety, but a certain amount of material stability and order in life was required to meet these needs. The need for love and affiliation was next highest on the ladder followed by the need for self esteem. To satisfy esteem needs self respect and a sense of achievement had to be felt. Finally, 'self actualisation' if fulfilled allowed a person to become all that he was capable of becoming. The extent to which individuals are able to forego fulfilment of some needs, and the interaction of needs was also considered by Maslow (see Fig. 5).

It will be apparent that there are some similarities in the last two approaches. The very ill patient suffering from an acute attack of asthma is very much concerned with the first of Virginia Henderson's identified needs 'to breathe' or Maslow's 'physiological needs'. Assessment of the patient at home will not be confined solely to the immediate problem but also later needs if perchance there is a further attack. In the intervening period the physiological, safety, and emotional (love and affiliation) wants of the patient and the relatives would be obvious. Much of the district nurse's time is spent in assisting the person to satisfy unmet 'physiological needs'. Criteria for what are considered to be basic needs vary considerably between different people. Gratification of the higher needs of those patients who are housebound or bedfast is often a great challenge and as with some aspects of physical care, other sources of help may be enlisted. District nurses will often be surprised at the tenacity and fortitude of patients in pursuing previous lifestyle.

REFERRAL OF PATIENTS TO THE DISTRICT NURSE

The first visit and overall assessment will be done by the District Nurse SRN.

The patient is central to the exercise of assessment although the district nurse begins collecting information and equipping herself in readiness for the first meeting from the time she receives the referral message. The message may contain basic details of name, age, address and any pertinent clinical background on a standard form from the hospital or another member of the primary care team, perhaps the receptionist, or it may be passed directly from one of these sources. On occasions the request may come from the patient or someone acting on the patient's behalf. The district nurse herself may sometimes identify a person she meets or hears about at a primary care team meeting, as a potential recipient of the district nursing service. According to the source and content of the referral note, the nurse uses her previous knowledge to decide if additional information is required and what equipment she may need before making her first visit. If a patient is being transferred home from hospital after extensive abdominal surgery and requiring a wound sinus to be irrigated or packed, a conversation with the ward sister will take place or perhaps a meeting arranged so that the finer points of nursing care can be ascertained. The passing of a nursing care plan from the hospital staff to the district nurse (and vice versa) is ideal for continuity of care. If the patient is referred from a member of the primary care team, records of the patient's history may be available. The health visitor or social worker may be asked about anything relevant, such as the patient's knowledge of his illness, or the probability of someone being in the house at the time of the nurse's visit. Occasionally the referral may come from the occupational health department of the patient's place of work, in which case the district nurse may wish to contact her colleague in occupational health.

It is sound policy for the nurse to have as many facts as are available to hand when making the first visit. Certain facts are essential for safe practice, the obvious one being the patient's medical diagnosis. Any diagnostic reports and any disabilities of the patient which might prevent him from responding to the nurses call, would hopefully also be known. While gaining this information other subjective information may be heard which may be helpful when meeting the patient. The nurse will probably wish to keep an open mind particularly if the patient has been presented in an unfavourable light. Such remarks may have been justified, but anticipation of difficulties can occasionally lead to their perpetuation. The overall assessment will be done by the District Nurse

(SRN) but the Enrolled District Nurse will be familiar with the process and contribute any developments observed by her.

INITIAL RELATIONSHIPS

Equipped with factual and subjective information the nurse will know what she hopes to achieve at the first visit.

A full assessment can only be done if the household is approached in an acceptable way and an atmosphere of trust is experienced by the patient and the nurse. Prior knowledge of the approximate time when the nurse can be expected helps to prepare the way for good relationships in a new household where the days routine has to be reorganized, even though this may be difficult to arrange. There is an element of the unknown even when the nurse is expected and the competent district nurse tunes in to the people and surroundings by showing courtesy, respect and interest while allowing the patient and family time to get to know who she is and the purpose of her visit. Genuine interest can usually be differentiated from an impersonal inquiry, followed by brusque unconvincing assurance. The direct look and smile of greeting may convey assurance of the patient's worth and the nurses willingness to listen to his problems.

Usually the patient and family will be expecting to have a long talk with the nurse at the first meeting, and if so the stage is set for a full nursing history to be taken. Obviously a patient waiting for his first injection may not wish to pour out his life story until after he has received his injection when there will be time to talk about future care. While the nurse is checking critical past history and observing clinical signs, (e.g. temperature, pulse, respiration and urine test, prior to giving a first gold injection for example), she will also be explaining her actions. The patient and others in the household will be noting the nurse's manner of approach when requesting a specimen of urine, work space or a place to wash her hands. Recognition of others present, and greeting them or their pets by name may help to cement relationships and open up lines of communication. Thus the patient's confidence in the nurse will be encouraged by the value she places upon his individual worth. The way will then be paved for further exchange of information.

The referral message does not always come from an informed source. A request from a neighbour to visit a frail elderly person in need of nursing help, may bring the nurse unexpectedly into contact with someone who has been hiding a fungating wound for some months. This person might accept some help at the first visit, but if the patient quickly shows signs of fatigue, the history can be built up gradually. Meantime the nurse would follow up any gaps in the medical or social history.

THE PATIENT AND FAMILY INTERVIEW

'The nursing interview . . . denotes any interaction either verbal or nonverbal, between a nurse and patient. . . . In this context, a bed-bath would take place within the framework of an interview'.[10]

All the incidental interaction which takes place between the district nurse and her patient has significance, but wherever possible a period should be devoted entirely to talking with the patient in a relaxed atmosphere and free from the distraction of 'doing'. The purpose of the interview is to gain as complete a picture of the person as possible. During the interview the patient will also be forming his views of the nurse as a person and as a representative of her profession.

The time required to take a formal nursing history may vary from twenty minutes to an hour or more. Whenever a patient is visited for the first time, certain information has to be obtained for the Kardex system, and for any nursing care plans which are to be left in the house. If the patient is too ill or unable to talk easily a relative may be asked to give the history but if this is so, unless it is contra-indicated by the patient's medical condition, he should be included in the conversation. The patient who has had a stroke and whose speech is affected may be very frustrated because he cannot answer for himself, but he would be even more agitated if he partly overheard what was being said about him in another room.

The nurse will find it helpful if she follows a similar pattern with each new patient. This ensures that essential areas are covered, although by picking up cues from the person's response, she will find it necessary to give more time to some aspects than others. Distress may be interpreted by her as a signal to pass on to another area in which the patient feels more comfortable or to pause and allow the patient or relative to decide whether they wish to continue on the same subject.

The district nurse will judge from the response she receives, and her nursing knowledge, just how much information it is necessary to have, and how much the patient is prepared to disclose about himself at the first meeting.

In any event there should not be a long period between the time of the first meeting and the completion of the nursing history. The minimum information gained at the first visit should be sufficient to ensure the patients identification, (name, age, address) and his safety, including the basic readings of T.P.R. B/P urinalysis, observation of general appearance and anything else pertinent to the care to be given would also be expected. Reciprocally the patient would expect to be given the nurse's name, where contact can be made in emergency, and the time of the next visit. An opportunity for the patient to also ask questions should be included. Attention is paid to all sources of information particularly that given by the patient. The referral message, previous health records, and consultation with other members of the primary health care team, the hospital ward sister, the consultant, or therapist may all be relevant when compiling a nursing history. Goals and plans of care will then be feasible.

DEFINING THE PROBLEM

The district nurses education equips her to apply problem solving techniques to her sphere of work. First the problem(s) have to be defined, and finding the right words to express patients problems is not always easy. Skill in picking up cues from unvoiced needs can be acquired. If the patient says he has a problem, the cause too will often be mentioned, which makes for ease of phraseology.

The most frequent nursing problems will be those connected with:

1. The daily living activities of eating, drinking, washing, dressing, elimination, sleeping positioning, and mobility.
2. The special senses.
3. Medication and treatment.

A closer look at these 'unmet needs' will often uncover more complex needs. There may be a number of reasons why a patient is not eating sufficiently. If this is 'due to nausea', it may be better to tackle the problem of nausea due to gastritis and follow this problem through, although inability to take an adequate diet may still be a valid problem for attention. Loss of appetite may also follow the habit of taking small infrequent meals stemming from a social or emotional cause such as poverty, or loss of recognition in the family. Jotting down all the possible problems helps the nurse to select from the initial assortment of interrelated problems those deserving priority in the subsequent action plans. Problems must be selected according to the criteria of urgency, greatest need, and the prospect of resources for their solution.

At this stage it is possible to frame aims and objectives of care which are realistic and acceptable to the patient and care-givers.

AIMS, GOALS AND PLANS OF CARE

Aims of care are general statements of the direction which the patient will follow and his eventual achievements or state of health.

Four examples of these are:

1. To recover maximum health (following influenza).
2. To achieve independence and mobility (within the limitations of his spasticity and the inconvenience of the household).
3. To regain full independence (following shock caused by burglary).
4. To maintain personal comfort continuing to take as active a part as possible in family life (despite disability).

The aims of care are overall statements which can only be achieved if more specific objectives or goals of care have been attained. Goals are more detailed and definitive than the general aim; they are statements of actions, behaviour or outcomes of patient care framed for each problem which are identified in the nurse's assessment.

A patient who has been transferred home from hospital after an uncomplicated appendicectomy would have the general aim of care, 'to return to full time work following appendicectomy'. His only 'unmet need' may be that he requires nursing help for 'removal of sutures'. If he is uncertain about his diet, or when to resume activities of heavy lifting or car driving, these problems and goals would need to be added to the list.

Table 3. Aims and goals of care.

Problem	Goal
Problem 1 Post-operative appendicectomy wound	Completely healed wound
Problem 2 Uncertain when he can resume heavy lifting and car driving	To become fully informed about progress and prospects

While the above may seem trivia it does perhaps illustrate that the second problem might be overlooked unless noted. The carefully considered action plan spells out the programme which the patient, nurse or relative is to follow in order to reach the desired goal.

There is therefore a logical sequence between:

The Patient's Problem	*Goal*	*Action*	*Evaluation*
	conditions and criteria	by whom and when	

A possible formula for goal setting which has been described by a number of writers can be recommended.[11] While there is some variation in their methods there is general agreement that the goal (and action plan) should include:

1. *The intended action* or outcome
2. The *performance* of the patient and or the performance of the person who is helping him.
3. The *criteria* by which this performance is to be measured.
4. The *conditions* (time, place, etc.) under which the performance/ behaviour is to take place.
5. The *consequence* of the results.

All patients cannot be cured, nor indeed can all problems be solved. Nevertheless, if the patient warrants a visit from the district nurse, some positive advantage to the patient is implied. Negative feelings are understandable when each new approach from the nurse meets with rebuttal or defeat. 'Goal setting' helps to change attitudes of 'therapeutic nihilism'.[12] The setting of short term goals is useful when nursing intervention is indicated but not immediately acceptable to the patient. If an elderly person has neglected his health for so long that he is socially isolated, a detailed assessment would obviously be desirable but the doctor and nurse may have to work towards this gradually. Meantime some acceptable short-term goals may be agreed.

District nurses invariably have a few patients within their caseload who are receiving periodic visits for supervision. These patients may

Table 4. Setting short-term goals

Problem	Goal	Action
Lack of interest in food	Restimulation of appetite	Daily discussion with the district nurse and the introduction of food supplements which will be obtained from . . .
Relectance to accept help with general hygiene and household tasks	To educate the patient towards a change of attitude	To introduce the patient to the health and social services available from the district nurse, general practitioner, and social worker. To try to make a decision about the need for future help in one week's time

have stable conditions, and the goal and plan of care may be designed to ensure that stability is maintained, and deviations from the expected course detected.

District nurses may be working with General Practitioners who have become accustomed to Problem Orientated Record Systems. This method which was pioneered by Lawrence Weed also focussed on patients problems.[13] Subjective information (that which the patient or relative volunteered) and objective information (that which the professional person observed, including clinical data) was assessed and planned for. This is also known as the Subjective Objective, Assessment, Plan Method of organizing and recording treatment and care. Problem lists can be amended as the occasion arises. An adaptation of this system for district nursing has been postulated by Dr. J.B. McIntosh. Where this is an agreed system used by general practitioners and district nurses their patients will doubtless benefit.

Earlier it was emphasized that 'the process' is *Patient Centred* and that the nurse works with the patient and family. There are occasions when the district nurse may find her aims of care conflicting with those which are acceptable to the patient. The extent to which the patient and family can be involved in the planning of care may be queried if the patient is mentally confused, or if the patients health values are different from those of the professional person. When meeting either of these eventualities professional integrity must not be abandoned while colluding with the patient in a plan which would endanger his health. Yet where the point at issue is not one of immediate life and death, there must of necessity be an element of choice left to the patient after the risks are known. No nurse would agree to a compromise in relation to a fire hazard, although in effect this cannot always be completely prevented, e.g. the patient who chooses to nod off to sleep in front of an unguarded fire at home, cannot be required by law to have a fireguard. The nurse however may be neglecting her duties if she has foreseen a danger and not recommended action. Educational aims related to the removal of long accustomed habits will cause the district nurse much heart searching when consulting and co-operating with the patient on these issues. There is a nicety of balance to be maintained between the liberty of the individual, and the professional responsibility of the district nurse. Society has expectations regarding the rights of the individual, and the conduct of the professional person. The professional person has a duty to herself, her patient and her profession.

Another point of conflict for the district nurse may be that the ideal model of care is not practical in terms of either the number of district nursing staff available or within time constraints. The acutely ill or severly disabled person may require nursing attention two to three hourly. Rehabilitation measures often depend upon frequent visits when new habits are being learned. The district nurse who is using 'the process' cannot avoid facing the totality of needs, whether she decides to programme more visits for herself, to identify the need for more staff or to seek alternative means of help for the patient.

The quality of nursing care may be adversely affected because problems allied to nursing are present such as inadequate laundry facilities or inadequate housing. Resources to meet such difficulties and the willingness of patients to press for their solution will vary. The previous criteria suggested of degree of urgency and the possibility of amelioration may be applied when deciding whether such problems are to be listed.

Lack of harmony within the family or within the person may give rise to many patients problems but unless these are openly identified by the persons concerned it will scarcely be acceptable to list such problems or incorporate their solutions in plans to be left in patients houses. If such problems can be phrased so that the patient's self image is preserved so much better. 'Days alone without activity are tedious' may be preferable to 'loneliness' which has connotations of personal inadequacies in relating to others. Similarly it may be acceptable to be 'concerned because of need to ask for frequent attention' but not to be 'unable to refrain from making frequent demands'. The nurse does not ignore these problems, nor does she set herself up as a counsellor par excellence, but she sifts the information for possible solutions. The psychological, sociological, ethical and legal implications of the options open will be considered in such complex situations. Where the patient is at risk of mental or physical abuse some record will need to be kept in the most appropriate place. (See Chapters 3 and 6.) Less serious problems of an emotional nature may be unspoken but understood between patient and nurse. Some action to relieve the non-articulated problem might still be included in the nursing plan. The most obvious one being 'Time for discussion (of progress)'.

This raises the question of the quantity and content of information to be left in the patient's house. It seems reasonable to leave the nursing care plan, if the patient and family are expected to follow its directions. Whether the problem list is also left in the house is a matter for local discussion and agreement between district nurse(s) and the nurse managers. The history sheet has served its initial purpose when the first problems have been identified but as this is the baseline it may be needed for future reference.

The nursing care plan and a progress sheet are the minimum essentials for continuity of care. As mentioned earlier there are advantages in framing goals which are linked with action plan.

Access to patients' records is being dealt with in Chapter 6, but brief comment on this and the form of the document is relevant here. If the nursing process is to improve the quality of nursing, a parallel improvement in the quality of records and communication documents is implied. The quality and content of any nursing record is determined by its purpose. Where it is local policy that nursing care plans and progress reports should be seen by all lay and professional helpers this will influence the detail which the district nurse will include. The progress report may contain or have attached to it messages to and from the patient, relative, doctor, health visitor, community psychiatric nurse. In the past the district nurse has been the only professional person to leave a progress report in the patients house. There is sound reason for this practice to continue, with the addition of the nursing care plan if the patient is to be increasingly informed about his own care. District nurses will have to decide whether the patient care plan and progress report is for their use alone, or should others beside the hitherto accepted general practitioner be invited to view and to contribute. A local policy recommending the latter could, if well thought out, have benefits for the patient. Some safeguards would need to be built in to the system to prevent abuse of confidentiality.

The expertise of the district nurse is nursing the patient in his home. Physical incapacity, or its predisposition is assumed by her presence although on occasions the actual physical care may be either of an advisory nature or anticipated at a later date. The value of her expertise may depend upon the help that is available to the patient from other professionals. In these circumstances the district nurse is acting as a co-ordinator. One would however expect that the nursing care plan agreed between the patient and the district nurse would clearly state the nurses actions; and not become solely the repository of those expected by, or from everyone else.

ADVANTAGES OF THE PROCESS IN CASELOAD MANAGEMENT

Using this systematic approach the district nurse is able to use her own time and resources and those of the nursing team more effectively. She is able to gain an estimate of nursing effectiveness by referring to patients nursing care plans. Justification for the employment of nursing staff will always be required and with the more detailed patient assessment a truer picture of patient dependency on nursing staff can be presented. Some of the dependency criteria used for hospital patients are not directly transferable to patients at home.[13] The amount of the district nurse's time given to the severely incapacitated patient at home is often determined more by the resources available in the family than the degree of incapacity of the patient. There is also some evidence that those who are most in need of help are not receiving the greatest attention.[14] Where two frail elderly people are living together their disadvantages may be compounded. Such information will be on record with the new system, and overall the district nurse would be in a position to prepare the case for or against more nursing resources to be directed to one household or to her total caseload. It would be possible for her to collate evidence at any time regarding such problems as nutritional deficiencies, skin lesions or mobility difficulties. The number of problems and the relationship of these to the patient, his resources and environment could be extracted from records.

Goals and plans of care not only act as incentives to the patient and staff, but can be used to estimate how much staff time will be required in the future. Where a plan includes a component of teaching this is less likely to be crowded out if a time for its evaluation is documented. This and other aspects of district nurses work will be more accessible, and thus more authoritative replies to questions about district nursing can be given.

Identification of nursing criteria will be promoted because the district nurse will have information to support her statements. This will not all be in the form of facts and figures but because she has studied both the patients and her own values she will be better able to present an informed view.

In differentiating nursing problems from those which may be more rightly solved by other community health, social or welfare workers, the district nurse may find that she has a wider contribution to make to the community. This may be in respect of local policies for health services but could relate to any community service.

Co-operation and communication points with colleagues and volunteers will be sharpened by the correct use of the nursing process. Co-operation between professionals of the statutory services is a foregone necessity. It is probable that in the last two decades of the twentieth century, with increasing emphasis being placed upon community self-help, the extent to which good neighbours and voluntary organizations provide support for patients will be greater. Acknowledgement for their support, combined with the limitations of community voluntary resources could be extracted from the nursing care plans.

Nursing may be more an art than a science. The sensitivity with which the nursing is delivered to the patient is an art to be acquired. The improved documentation of nursing will help to clarify the scientific basis of district nursing within nursing. District nurses have always been ready to accept responsibility and the nursing process provides a system of management with in-built accountability to the patient, to the nurse herself and to her profession.

REFERENCES

1. Panel of Assessors for District Nurse Training.
   Curriculum in District Nursing for State Registered Nurses and Registered General Nurses. December 1978.
2. McINTOSH, J.B. Record Keeping – a boon or a bind? *Nursing Mirror*, July 1978.
3. Community Health Nursing. (1974). Report of a WHO Expert Committee. *Technical Report, Series 558*.
4. A working group of the Scottish National Nursing and Midwifery Consultative Committee. A new concept of nursing. *Nursing Times*, April 1978.
5. HARGREAVES, I. The Nursing Process. *Nursing Times*. August 28th, 1975.
6. KRATZ, C.R. (1979) Ed. *The Nursing Process*. London: Baillière Tindall.
7. Rcn Working Party (1980). *Primary Health Care Nursing: A Team Approach*.
8. HENDERSON, V. (1968). *Basic Principles of Nursing Care*. International Council of Nurses.
9. MASLOW, A.H. (1943). A Theory of Motivation. *Psychological Review, Vol. 50*, p. 390–6. As abridged in *Management and Motivation*, ed. Vroom and Beci (1970). Harmondsworth: Penguin.
10. MURRAY, J.B. (1963). Self Knowledge and the Nursing Interview. *Nursing Forum* 2(L), 69–78.
11. GLOVER MAYERS, M. (1972). *A systematic approach to the Nursing Care Plan*. New York: Appleton Century Crofts/New York Division of Prentice Hall.
    DAVIES, A.D.M. & CRISP, A.G. (July 1980) Setting performance goals in geriatric nursing. *Journal of Advanced Nursing*. London: Blackwell Scientific Publications.
    KUSHLICK, A., BLUNDEN, R., HOMER, D. & SMITH, J. (1975). *The Handicapped Person in the Community*. Open University Post Experience Course, Unit 9.
12. WEED, L.L. (1970). *Medical Records, Medical Education and Patient Care*. Press of Cape Western Reserve University.
    McINTOSH, J.B. Record keeping — a boon or a bind? *Nursing Mirror*, July 6th, 13th and 20th, 1978.
13. RHYS HEARN, C. Evaluation of patients nursing needs. *Nursing Times*, October 1974.
14. PASKER, P., THOMAS, J.P.R. & ASHLEY, J.S. (1975). *Study of Geriatric Population*. North East Essex.
    KRATZ, C.R. (1978). *Care of the Long Term Sick in the Community*. Edinburgh: Churchill Livingstone.

CHAPTER 3

Caseload Management

Caseload management is the planned use of time. It is complicated because the number of actual and potential patients will always outstrip the capacity of the service to meet all the demands made upon it, and this situation is not likely to be remedied in the foreseeable future. Some rationing is inevitable, but the basis upon which this takes place is often ill-defined and haphazard. Hospitals when overwhelmed with work adjust their admissions procedure, and in times of acute staff shortage shut down wards and departments. The district nursing service must accept all referrals initially and then must decide what work can be safely managed with the existing resources. All advice on caseload management recommends the selection of priorities, but is less specific about what can be left undone. It is useful to distinguish between caseloads and work-loads. A heavy caseload does not necessarily imply a heavy workload. Many patients may not need prolonged visiting — if they are given planned intensive care initially with the appropriate health teaching they may achieve their optimum independence within days or weeks and then be ready for discharge or regular short supervisory visits. However, a few patients without supporting relatives may require a lot of work to be done for them with little prospect of its reduction during their lifetime.

Not all visits are equally useful. Some supervisory visits may be too infrequent to effect any improvement in the patient's state of health, some may even fail to halt deterioration that could have been prevented. Some visits degenerate into social calls without retaining any planned therapeutic purpose. Some visits are very difficult to regulate, recently some families have taken legal advice when visiting has been reduced claiming entitlement to such routine care as blanket bathing for their elderly relatives. Such pressures make it very necessary for the nurse not only to know but to be able to explain and have recorded the grounds on which she gives care to one patient and not to another.

When responsible for a caseload it is necessary to estimate the balance of work that will result in the greatest good for the greatest number of patients. To do this it is necessary to monitor regularly how much time is spent in each of several groups of activities, as well as how much is spent with each individual patient. Activities that need to be balanced in the management of any caseload include:

1. Caring for those who are sick and unable to care for themselves, or in teaching and supervising others who are providing such care.

2. Observing patients in their particular environment. Some observations will relate to the patient's illness, such as vital signs, changes in symptoms, reactions to drugs, the possibility of fracture or dislocation, or they may be observations of the patient's attitude to his disease, of the competence and dependability of the family in their caring role, judging whether they understand the treatment, the prognosis, or the changes in lifestyle necessary for recovery or rehabilitation.

3. Teaching and counselling with families and groups, particularly those directed to increasing the families' capacity to cope with their own problems and to become more self directing.

4. Supporting individuals and groups as they cope with their problems. This may be standing by the family of a patient with a long-term illness, listening to the disappointment and resentment of a severely handicapped person, or just being available on the telephone to the daughter of a mentally disturbed patient.

5. Carrying out treatments, diagnostic tests and other investigations in the surgery, health clinic or the patient's home.

6. Integrating and co-ordinating the various services needed by a particular patient, undertaking the reporting referral and the interpretation of his condition essential for effective care.

7. Participating in general staff matters such as:
(a) training and supervising students
(b) compiling statistics
(c) organizing and managing special clinics such as those for patients with varicose veins
(d) developing health education projects
(e) initiating and assisting in research

This list gives only a crude measure but it is probably more useful than simply dividing the work into home care, surgery duties, travelling time and office work.

It may eventually be decided as a matter of policy that too much time is being spent on any particular activity, but generally it is better to adjust the balance between them thereby conserving a diverse and interesting workload as well as utilizing a range of nursing skills. This will also offer a service that is more likely to be justly allocated to those who need it.

There is always a difference between the patients who get priority treatment and those who are said to be priority cases, nor are either group necessarily those the nursing staff would think should have the first call on their time. Kratz, in her study of stroke patients nursed at home,[1] found that patients who were not going to get better were undervalued by the district nurses. It is necessary to ensure that all patients are assessed accurately and are given a just proportion of the nurse's time and attention. Priority is often given to patients who at the time may not be the most deserving. They may for example be those who:

1. Are particularly vocal in demanding service.
2. Suffer from cancer.
3. Have terminal illness.
4. Are particularly favoured by the medical staff, either because of personality, status or for clinical interest.
5. Have certain problems that are socially inacceptable such as lack of hygiene, bedfastness, faeceal incontinence or gross urinary incontinence. These are quickly referred by doctors, neighbours, health visitors, social workers and clergy as being problems that district nurses should be able to remedy or at least modify.
6. Some patients and some nursing situations are in themselves attractive, and to them the nurses readily respond. Frequently they are optimistic patients who have a buoyant attitude to life, whatever their prognosis. Those who cooperate well with their nurses and those who respond to treatment.

It should always be remembered that care given to any particular patient is done at the expense of others, therefore it is important to be as objective and as free from bias as possible when deciding upon the priorities of the caseload.

Every history taken should be presented in such a way that the problems of dysfunction and nursing needs are easily identified and the nurse should give an opinion about the resources needed to solve the one and meet the other. It is important to state that these opinions should be modified during the course of treatment.

Case records should give summaries of care at frequent intervals and whenever there is marked change in the patient's condition. The summaries should include:

1. A recapitulation of nursing needs and the short term aims.
2. An outline of the social situation and other agencies involved.
3. The frequency of visits needed and the chances of success which may be expressed in terms of treatment completed, rehabilitation, or the family being able to cope.

The nursing teams together with the general practitioners should evaluate the work in the light of all the summaries and together endorse or modify the programmes of those patients whose treatment is complex or those who require a lot of nursing time.

The nursing teams should meet together with the team leader to discuss:

1. The priorities that they see in their workloads.
2. The reasons for and against the discharging of certain patients.
3. Methods of achieving adequate patient care by other means than direct nursing service, i.e. use of volunteers, or combination of voluntary and statutory services. Provision of appliances or apparatus to increase mobility.

This exercise in caseload management can be used simply to measure the situation at any time, and effect small changes in the team's priorities. This may be seen as its sole purpose. However, if it is continued systematically month by month the constant reappraisal of priorities monitoring the effectiveness of work, and the reallocation of resources provides evidence of the need for a change in manpower levels and nursing policies as circumstances change. The exercise will show:

1. Which problems and activities are actually receiving the highest priority in terms of time spent upon them.

2. The discrepancy between what is said about what is done for patients and what is actually done, for example how comprehensive is the nursing care given, how appropriate is the health teaching and what is the nature of the support given to families.

3. The factors that mitigate against using the nursing process properly. For instance this may not be shortage of time, or of staff but reluctance

on the part of nurses to take detailed nursing histories when this involves asking awkward questions.

4. The need to redefine priorities regularly and bring them into open debate with doctors, as well as with middle and top nursing management.

Several principles of caseload management will be decided after staff consultation. Some may be enshrined in the policy laid down by health authorities, some are determined locally by the primary health care team. Inevitably what is done for any particular patient is decided when the nurse visits. It will depend upon the urgency of need, the vulnerability of patient and family and the competing claims of the other patients to be seen that day. There is no blueprint for assessing relative need that can be written into a general textbook: only guidelines can be drawn. These guidelines present some of the factors that may pertain in any set of circumstances and may act as an *aide mémoire* when making decisions, nothing more.

HOW PATIENTS COME INTO DOMICILIARY CARE

Patients are referred to the district nursing service from many sources, most come from the general practitioners, some are sent by the hospitals. Social workers from both statutory and voluntary organizations may request help for their clients; friends, neighbours and the family may recognize need and approach the nurse directly. There are patients who come to seek the nurse's help themselves and some who must be sought out by the nurse, such as the vulnerable in cold weather or the bronchitics in fog.

In order to get in touch with those who may need care the nursing staff must be prepared to make themselves known, and describe what they can do in certain circumstances, to patients in the practice or residents of the neighbourhood in which she works. It is useful if the nurse works in the surgery during the doctor's consulting hours so that she is known by sight to some patients before they need her services. She should be able and willing to speak to neighbourhood groups about the work of the primary health care team. This not only reassures the potential patient it will be well done but it helps to encourage a sympathetic and compassionate attitude to the sick, the aged and the infirm in the locality. Many voluntary workers and home helps are recruited by enthusiastic people already involved in caring who are willing to share their experiences and talk realistically not only about their work but also of the satisfactions that come from working with patients.

GATHERING INFORMATION

It is essential when accepting new work to gather enough information. It is easy to overlook some of the important factual information if the caller is agitated and whoever receives the call does not have a framework for collecting such identification data as: name, age, address, name of general practitioner by whom referred, diagnosis, problems and treatment. Such telephone conversations as:

> 'Will you come to Mrs Smith she has fallen out of bed?'
> 'Where does Mrs. Smith live?'
> 'Next door to me.'
> 'Where do you live?'
> 'In the house with the yellow door', or worse still, 'Next door to Mrs Smith.'

are not uncommon and occasionally the nurse tired after a heavy day can ring off before she knows where to find poor Mrs Smith.

Whenever possible a diagnosis should be obtained. This will vary in precision according to who makes the approach to the nurse, but always when treatment is prescribed the nurse should be sure that she knows enough about the patient's condition and the nature of the tasks she is being asked to perform. Drugs and applications should be familiar to her, when they are not or the prescribed dose is different from usual they should be checked directly with the doctor and, if possible, a written confirmation of dosage and drug should be given to her. Whenever the nurse has reason to question the instructions given to her a note to this effect should be attached to the case notes.

The nurse needs adequate information if errors are to be avoided and the patient's safety ensured. Some patients, those with infected wounds for example, or a contageous disease, will be nursed at such a time when they are least danger to the patient who may be next on the work list. There are also times when the nurse needs to know for her own protection the exact nature of the underlying condition as well as the treatment she is being asked to give. An ulcer that is syphilitic in origin or a bronchitis that is tubercular may well require different techniques of work from those which are less infective and will be visited at a time of day when the nurse is not overtired or hungry.

It is not realistic to expect detailed or personal information to be passed to the nurse if she is not available to receive it. Messages left with a clerk or secretary should be entered in a book or on a card in such a way that essential facts are recorded, and a phone number should be taken so that the nurse can ring back and speak to the professional person making the referral, clarifying any points about which she is uncertain and thereby avoiding any misunderstanding or error.

Whenever there is a complex message to be passed it should be passed directly between the professional workers concerned either by the spoken or the written word. It may be expedient to use the telephone for a message but it may be safest to write down an instruction, and in some cases it may be better for the district nurse to visit the patient in the ward, to discuss with the ward sister the methods of treatment devised for the patient's comfort and safety. The district nurse must always insist upon adequate and safe communication when treatment is either started or changed.

Post-operative patients surrounded by gleaming trolleys, bowls and instruments think of their irrigations and dressings as minor operations, it is helpful for them to see the district nurse before they are discharged and hear from her how the principles of their care will not change though the procedure will be carried out in their bathroom or kitchen. Another group of patients who experience anxiety before discharge are the paraplegic patients who are being transferred home from a special unit. In hospital they have learned to be independent, when they come home they must carry on the same routine as far as possible. They need to know whether the district nurse will be able and willing to work with them or whether they will be expected to conform to her way of working and perhaps be subjected to an imposed regime more suited to a patient with a degenerative disease than a physically rehabilitated adult.

The nurse acccepting a patient from hospital or any other source has certain responsibilities to the patient's general practitioner. These include:

1. Notifying the doctor of the patient's referral and his condition on discharge.

2. Notifying him of other workers that may be involved with his patient.

3. Warning him, if it seems likely that the patient or his family do not understand about the treatment needed, or are unwilling to carry out the instructions given.

4. Supplying him with comprehensive reports of the patient's progress, and timely requests for the dressings and drugs that are needed.

THE FIRST VISIT

The pattern of work set at the first visit is particularly important. What is said, what is used, how much help is sought or accepted, and the quality of the teaching that is given will determine the cooperation of the patient and his family on future occasions. There is considerably more inclination at the beginning of treatment to cooperate and learn from the nurse. When what she has said makes good sense, and when her attitude is one of come and learn, patient and family will experience comfort and soon feel secure enough to become involved with the nursing care.

Preparation

How can the nurse prepare for a visit in such a way as to be able to share her work with the patient and family? She must meet anxieties and their need for knowledge, as well as create a nursing environment, and start the complicated task of history taking. There must be an adequate system of referral and, wherever possible, access for the nurse to the medical records of the family. The more knowledge the nurse can accrue, the more practical preparations she can make. If in doubt it is better to go to a patient armed with bed protection and incontinence pads only to find the patient up and able to go to the toilet. To arrive without equipment when it is needed is to start at a disadvantage. To meet or be seen to be able to meet a practical need is reassuring to the patient and to know she is well prepared gives the nurse confidence. Freedom from anxiety enables the nurse to concentrate on the patient's problems and take advantage of every teaching opportunity that might arise.

Interaction

Important though the history taking is, care must be taken that natural and spontaneous interaction is not inhibited by the need to gather information, or give instruction. Such topics as care of the patient, care and storage of drugs, observations to be made and the possible consequences of any prescribed treatments should be introduced into a discursive conversation rather than stated as a sequence of rules to be obeyed. Furthermore, the conversation should be so directed that within a few minutes the patient or care-giver is encouraged to repeat the important teaching back to the nurse. This should not be as an answer to a direct question but as a response to an indirect query or remark.

It is often possible to help those taught to incorporate an idea, and indeed if they believe that they have though of it themselves so much the better. Patients and their families need their confidence built up. This is done by using all their resources, physical, intellectual and emotional. They should be helped to accept professional help as a complement to their own contribution, not as something better but different. It should be seen as a new perspective that can enrich their caring, never a reason for their withdrawal.

Organization

Practically it is advisable to make a definite statement of how you wish the work to be carried out, where and with what equipment. Managing in an inadequate space with poor lighting, or with limited hot water for instance on a first visit is sometimes interpreted by the family as normal practice and it is very difficult at a subsequent visit to raise the environmental standards, or insist on different resources being made available. This is particularly important when the first visit is undertaken by a relief nurse and the regular staff have to take over on the second or third visit. Unless good practice has been initiated the quality of care is much more variable, not only in the facilities available, but in the family's commitment to caring and their willingness to try out new ideas. They also pay less attention to the health education component of the visit if they have not from the very first experienced combined caring and teaching.

FREQUENCY OF VISITING

One of the first questions relatives will want answered is how often the nurse will call and how much will she do when she comes. This will depend upon:

1. The patient's physical, emotional and social make up.
2. The specific condition he suffers from, the impairment of function that results from it, and the degree to which it inhibits the individual's ability to lead a normal life.
3. Who cares for the patient.
4. In what sort of environment, either emotional or structural, does the caring take place.

There are however certain conditions in which a patient is likely to require more frequent visiting.

1. The patient in the terminal stages of disease with acute pain. In these circumstances as many as three or four visits may be paid daily. The need for nursing care, the administration of drugs, the support of the relatives seldom pose any problems for the nurses directly concerned. They are generally pleased to get involved in the social and emotional

problems of the household as well as the nursing care. Their colleagues who are not concerned with the particular patient but who in consequence carry a heavier workload will not usually question intensive work with the dying, regarding it as reasonable and not likely to last for very long.

2. The patient who is in danger of developing pressure sores should be visited twice a day unless there is very competent and reliable help in the household.

3. Patients with gross incontinence are generally deserving of a second visit during the day as the relatives are already taxed by the extra washing and the problems of drying and airing bedding in bad weather are very tiring.

4. Patients for whom the treatment prescribed needs to be given more than once a day.

5. Patients with discharging wounds, particularly when a drainage tube has been inserted, may not be comfortable if left for twenty-four hours unattended.

6. Patients should be visited within the hour if they have had a substantial haemorrhage, and revisited four hours after that if possible.

7. Patients with an unexplained rise in temperature should be revisited within twelve hours as should any patient with a marked change in pulse rate, or rate of respiration.

8. A diabetic patient presenting with an acute infection should be revisited particularly when glucose has to be substituted for his normal diet.

9. The depressed patient or care-giver should be revisited in the majority of cases.

10. In all cases of unexpected deterioration.

In many of these cases where the nurse returns because of an unexplained change she will have sought medical opinion and the follow-up visit may be planned to coincide with that of the doctor.

While there is not usually much hesitation in visiting a cancer patient several times daily, twice daily visits to the long-term sick are regarded differently. When a group of nurses are assessing the need to visit a patient with rheumatoid arthritis or multiple sclerosis both in the morning and in the late afternoon, they may be starting on a commitment that could last many years. Yet the reluctance to visit frequently over acute phases of illness can lead to the condition resolving at a greater degree of dependency than might have been the case had more care been given in the correct proportions initially.

When nursing care is delegated to the patient, a family member or a neighbour, they must be entitled to relief from time to time. The diabetic patient who hates giving herself insulin might reasonably ask for the nurse to visit once a week or one week in five in order to give her a rest from the anxiety of giving her injection into her leg or her abdomen. The relative or neighbour who puts a patient back to bed each night may welcome a night off occasionally, or a break in order to go away. Such requests should be taken seriously as the relative who knows that she can expect help when she needs it will be more likely to be able to cope with months of demanding and sometimes heavy work.

There is considerable difference in the capacities of relatives, so the nurse must carefully assess the reality of the care that is being given. Willingness is not always the same as competence. The type of neighbourhood, the family and social networks enjoyed by the patient and the quality of the bonds that are forged between patient and care-giver are all important factors in determining the interval between visits.

There is a difference between the hygiene patterns met with in various households. It is not easy to judge the frequency of bathing, hairwashing, changing clothes or bed linen that is normal for any family, although there are some cultural influences and social class patterns that can be recognized. There is a marked difference in attitudes to washing all over as a substitude for bathing between people who have always had a hot water supply and central heating and those who grew up in houses where hot water for baths was only available occasionally and a kettle of water was usually all that was available. Where it is local policy for the sake of safety to wash or blanket bath rather than to help patients into the bath, those who have always been used to a daily bath may feel very deprived. Showers are becoming more common but are still not acceptable to some older patients, and they are not likely to be found in all homes for many years.

When caring takes place intermittently, that is two or three times a week or less frequently, there is need for careful record keeping so that there is a comprehensive pattern of care. Shorter frequent visits are often an economy in time providing the patient's home is in the centre of the district. Where much travelling is involved it is better to visit less frequently, all other things being equal. If, as is usually the case, the objective in caring is to promote independence the short, frequent visit allows more participation by the patient without the fatigue that accompanies longer and more comprehensive visits. There is very little nursing care that cannot be divided into several, smaller tasks. It is important to gauge the right amount to do for any particular patient so that the essentials are covered, and comprehensive care is achieved within a planned span of visits so that a just allocation of the time is possible between the various patients' competing needs.

DURATION OF DEPENDENCY

Deciding how frequently to visit is not a once a month or even once a week activity but a dynamic process that takes place at each visit. There is a danger associated with overvisiting and that is that the nurse may make the patient more dependent than necessary by taking over decision making that should properly be left with the patient. The elderly who have little self confidence will sometimes be quite happy to have the nurse tell them what they should do, what to eat, how they should exercise and even what television programmes they would enjoy.

Tasks too can be undertaken by the nurse because she does them better or more quickly than the patient or relative. This can do considerable harm. There is a temptation to want to bring patients all possible help, but bringing in the service of a home help or meals-on-wheels too soon may deprive an elderly woman of an interest. She may not need to go out to the shops to buy food and consequently lose the one opportunity each day to speak to someone, and to see other people going about their business. The right time to introduce services or to take over some function that the patient has done for himself is when the danger associated with the lack of hygiene or lack of nutrition due to his failing capacity is greater than the loss of independence.

There is a further danger, that of giving too little help. The patient who needs intensive care to achieve even partial independence may become chronically dependent if he is only given intermittent care. Patients who remain on the caseload indefinitely, neither improving nor deteriorating are frequently those for whom the original care plan was faulty.

There are secondary gains in long term illness. The elderly sick generally enjoy the nurse's visits and quickly they will establish them as a social event rather than professional visits which have as an objective moving towards independence. They will not want to do anything that will justify the nurse closing the case, and this sometimes includes recovering.

Illness is generally regarded as interesting. Patients can command, even for a short time, the undivided attention of doctors and nurses. Most enjoy the contact with professional people who are themselves interesting and at least locally hold positions of some prestige.

The major nursing endeavour should be directed towards making independence more attractive than dependence. The nurse must endeavour to make the social and emotional environment more supportive as well as concentrating upon the general rehabilitation programme that is an integral part of most care plans.

It is essential to lose patients from the caseload in order to have time for new patients. Some patients will recover, some will die, some will be able to manage with family support. If the nurse is unable to clear enough time to take new work it is often useful to ask a colleague to visit for her and reassess her more chronic patients. It may never be possible to discharge some patients who have become dependent, but such a reassessment may well reveal that if different action had been taken earlier more independence could have been achieved. Every nursing problem should be analysed at two levels, first in relation to the patient's individual treatment plan, and secondly in order to learn how to manage such problems better in future.

THE CARE OF DRUGS

Important observations are made by the district nurse when patients are having drug therapy at home. She must be alert to the variety of substances prescribed, where they are kept and how regularly they are taken. She must be able to recognize drug intolerance, the side effects of drugs used and the secondary symptoms that arise as a result of the medication.

There are particular dangers for the patients on drug therapy at home, for instance, the diabetic patient who is always slightly confused in the morning will not be able to split a tablet accurately and take only half, nor will he find it easy to take one tablet on alternate days without someone to help him. All drugs have side effects. Some are tolerable in the short term but used for a long period they give rise to greater discomfort than the symptoms they are supposed to relieve. Dryness of the mouth embarrasses those wearing dentures and makes speaking difficult. In a stroke patient a dry mouth can hinder rehabilitation by hindering the re-education of his cheek muscles, which is necessary if the patient is to be able to hold his dentures in place firmly enough to eat a proper meal. It also interferes with speech therapy. Sedation in the elderly may cause nocturnal confusion and incontinence. When elderly patients have several drugs prescribed for different conditions the side effects may be masked, or seen as symptoms of yet another disease requiring more medication. Drugs are absorbed at different rates by different people. With ageing and developing disease the metabolism and excretion of drugs may be impaired.

Another problem associated with drug therapy is the difficulty patients have following the instructions that are given to them. There is evidence to support the theory that very little information given by doctors is heeded by their patients. With the elderly the risk is increased by impaired hearing and faulty concentration. The nurse must make a plan with her elderly patients so that they know exactly what they should take, at what time and in what manner. It is sometimes helpful if the tablets are set out in special containers or labelled with symbols indicating the time they should be taken.

Some patients hold quite large stocks of drugs and furthermore they often know what would be the lethal dose. The nurse should realise the temptation these drugs represent to the depressed patient or harrassed relative. They may have been accumulated because the doctor prescribes liberally, or deliberately collected over a few weeks. Not all patients who accumulate drugs are suicidal, many patients never think about taking their own lives, but others find that peace of mind comes with the certain knowledge that they could do so should the situation become unbearable. The suspicion that the patient is accumulating drugs is one that should be shared between members of the caring team, and all professional visitors should monitor the patient's behaviour, counselling as appropriate. It is possible to prevent the impulsive action, that is a cry for help, by timely intervention. The patient who has thought through his problems carefully and plans to take an overdose will probably hide his intention from the most vigilant team.

Relatives have as much opportunity as the patient to collect drugs. It is essential therefore that the nurse watches for signs of undue stress in those who care for the patient. When scheduled drugs are prescribed the nurse should advise on their storage and if she is worried about emotional tensions in the household she may be wise to check the drugstore regularly. Drugs may be taken accidentally as well as intentionally. Where there are young children in the home all poisonous substances must be locked away out of their reach.

When the nurse is responsible for the administration of drugs in the course of the patient's illness she must keep a record of the drugs supplied, the date and time of their administration, the type of infection and the site selected. All entries should be signed with a full signature.

REGULATIONS GOVERNING THE HOLDING OF SCHEDULED DRUGS[2]

The regulations governing the prescribing and holding of supplies of scheduled drugs rest on three principles.[3]

1. That only authorized people may be in possession of drugs. There is a list of authorized people including:

> A duly qualified medical practitioner and the person for whom a drug has lawfully been prescribed by a registered medical practioner.
> A district nurse is *not* included in the list. She is therefore *not* permitted to have custody of a scheduled drug.

2. A person may not supply or offer to supply any drug, either to or for any person, including himself, unless authorized. A doctor who requires scheduled drugs for the purpose of his practice may obtain them from either a retail chemist, who is an unauthorized seller of poisons, or a wholesale dealer who is licensed by the Home Office to supply such drugs.

3. Drugs prescribed for the treatment of one patient may not be diverted to other patients or to the general need of the medical practice.

THE DISPOSAL OF DRUGS

When a nurse finds surplus drugs in the house she should try to persuade the person for whom they were prescribed to destroy them. As the drugs belong to the patient he may if he chooses keep them; he may not pass them to anyone else. As there is a risk of accidental poisoning or drug abuse if unneeded drugs are kept, the Home Office urges the destruction of all scheduled drugs.[4]

When the patient has died, the nurse, with the consent of the house-holder, should destroy the drugs still in the house whether they are opened or unopened, by burning or by pouring down the toilet.[5] The nurse should make a written statement as to the nature and amount of the drugs destroyed and obtain, if at all possible, the signature of another person who witnessed the destruction.

The drugs have been prescribed for the patient. The relatives are not authorized to have custody of them or supply them to anyone else. Neither the doctor nor the nurse is permitted to receive drugs from an unauthorized person.

PROBLEMS EXPERIENCED BY CERTAIN PATIENTS

CHILD PATIENTS

There are certain problems specific to children which may influence the amount and type of care given and the time at which it is given.

1. Disease processes differ according to age. A virus infection in an adult may pass unnoticed, in a school child it may pass as a cold. In a two-year-old the same virus may cause acute bronchitis and in a very young infant it may cause pneumonia or even bronchitis. Therefore the younger the child the more frequently should its condition be assessed.

2. Even after infancy the majority of communication with children is non-verbal. The child frequently sees and understands much more than the adults around realize. The knowledge of cancer, for example, often comes to the child from the adult's reactions rather than from what is said.

3. There is a need to woo the cooperation of the parents of a sick child. The more serious the diagnosis the greater are the parents' problems and their anxieties can come between them and other helpers. If the mother can feel confidence in the primary health care team this will help the child. If she regards the nurse and the treatment with fear and apprehension this will be transmitted to the young patient. Children should be visited by appointment early in the morning list so that the child can be assured that by a certain time each day treatment will be over. This minimized the strain of anticipation which always accompanies uncomfortable treatments.

4. A child belongs to a family and is an interdependent part relating to the whole. Socially, emotionally and physically the small child has a particular relationship with his mother, and generally she has special need of him. It is necessary in the home to nurse them both together, encouraging the mother to hold the child in the way that will bring him most comfort. It is seldom helpful for the nurse to take over the comforting role from the mother, although she may feel she should in order to atone for the hurt she is inflicting. The mother sometimes needs to be helped to feel only for the child and to disregard her own feelings about the treatment or about the child's behaviour. The mother who is embarrassed by the child who acts badly throughout his treatment may overcheck the child's outburst, thus turning the nurse and other caregivers into bogey men who cause hurt.

5. There is always need for health teaching at a visit to a child. The nurse will seize the opportunity to explain the advantages of immuniza-

tion, and screening for metabolic disorders. She will notice and get treatment for a squint. She will be aware of hazards in the environment always promoting safety measures.

6. The child is different at each stage of development. The characteristics of each stage should be known and revised before visiting. The nurse may have to follow the progress of a handicapped child through several stages of growth, as well as pay visits to children in any particular phase of development. This is a task which should be shared with the health visitor.

7. A comprehensive approach to nursing children must include awareness of the emotional as well as the physical effects of illness. The nurse must recognize the part played by poor social conditions in the origins of physical, mental, emotional and educational problems. A preventitive as well as a curative approach to the nursing care of a child may confer benefits that will last throughout his lifetime.

8. She will always be aware of the possibility of neglect or cruelty, and remain sensitive to inconsistencies between what is said and what is observed. The mother who while speaking words of comfort does not smile, the explanation about bruising that does not tally, the child whose face is drawn with pain and fear but who does not cry or protest. These signs should be carefully noted.

There is in each area a policy to be followed when neglect or cruelty is suspected. If the nurse is worried about a child she should seek the advice of a senior nursing colleague immediately.

PATIENTS SUFFERING FROM CANCER

There is still a great deal of fear in households and in the community that a patient who has cancer will have a very difficult last illness. Some do not, however all have considerable mental stress from the time the diagnosis is made to the end of their lives. This distress can be lessened if communication between professionals and patient is clear and unambiguous.

Much delay in reporting symptoms is caused by fear, months may elapse before patients pluck up courage to seek advice, and delay often increases the subsequent stress and suffering. District nurses, particularly those working in the surgeries, are often the first person to hear of strange symptoms that the patient wants investigated yet hesitates to ask about. Direct and indirect cancer education is one of the major responsibilities of the nurse. Seven danger signals that, if they persist, should be reported to the doctor are:

1. Unusual bleeding or discharge.
2. A lump or thickening in the breast or elswhere.
3. A sore that does not heal.
4. A change in bowel or bladder habits.
5. Indigestion or difficulty in swallowing.
6. Hoarseness or cough.
7. Change in a wart or mole.

Prevention

This includes:

1. Health screening clinics.
2. Smoking clinics.
3. Cytology tests.
4. Health screening at work.

Much fear is of treatment, hospitals, operations, radio therapy injections. The aim of the team of care-givers should always be to make the treatment of each patient as easily and as well understood as possible so that patients and relatives give a reassuring account of it to their friends and relations.

The patient has a great need of short term goals set by doctor, nurse and family. They should be as reassuring and encouraging as possible such as, sleeping better at night by the end of the week, less nausea by the end of the month.

The relatives often are fearful, sometimes their fears are groundless, but they are a manifestation of the guilt felt about the patient's deterioration. The best help relatives can receive is regular and genuine involvement in the responsibility of caring, not by giving them little jobs to do, but by taking them into the confidence of the nursing team and involving them in the decision taking. The use of technical terms used in professional conversations should be explained so that it is seen as an accurate form of communication, rather than a screen behind which care-givers can hide.

There is something about malignancy which we all find difficult to face in ourselves and in our patients. We look away, hesitate and talk about inflamation and ulcers. We do not help the patient by denying what he suspects, indeed we isolate him and may make him afraid to ask again. Most importantly *evasion* destroys trust.

For the patient who is dying peace and comfort is important. Each symptom should be dealt with as it arises, and if it cannot be abolished it can perhaps be eased. Kindliness and quiet competence is the essential ingredient of caring.

Wilkes[6] found that of the ten major symptoms experienced in patients in terminal illness pain is the most persistently reported. This must be attributed to several factors, including inadequate drug therapy. Fear, loneliness, and lack of personal support can reduce the effectiveness of the drugs prescribed. Breathlessness, nausea and vomiting can in some cases be relieved by drugs. Other symptoms may include incontinence, insomnia, confusion, anorexia, depression and anxiety.

Communication is important. The follow up of patients depends upon co-ordinated record keeping. The patient and his family need to have access to the hospital staff for consultations, as well as their general practitioner. The hospital needs information about the patient's home, the family support, the age of the caring relatives. The nursing team needs to know what help is available from the statutory and voluntary services. All need to know and understand the patient as a person to recognize his moods, what he is thinking about his condition, the amount of pain he experiences and the level of his anxiety.

Frequently it is difficult to tell when the patient comes to realize that he has a malignant growth and that he will die shortly. Realization comes gradually. Sometimes relatives are told what the diagnosis and prognosis is and carry this burden alone, trying to protect the patient who is likely to suspect even if his fears have never been confirmed. There is always stress in a situation where those involved do not know what to expect or for how long they will have to manage the work and the emotional tension. Families expect grief and anxiety to accompany terminal illness but they rarely expect the resentment, the escape into self deception and the false hopes that from time to time they and the patient experience when the truth is recognized. This feeling of resentment, which may be quite aggressive, and fear should be freely expressed to the nurse. When it can never be shared it is very hard to bear and may lead to relatives giving up their involvement in caring shortly before the patient dies. When this happens the guilt that they experience complicates their recovery from the bereavement and may remain with them all through their lives.

HELPING THE BEREAVED

Death and bereavement threaten and disturb us. When things threaten us we have defence mechanisms that come into play to ward off the impact of the reality of what is happening. We have both conscious and unconscious ways of avoiding the fact of bereavement. We do not know what to say. We tend to use the language of avoidance when we speak of death. We say someone has passed away, for example. We do not talk about the effect the death has on those left and we try to stop their tears. We try to think that there is a solution to the very complex problem. We tend to prescribe rather than counsel and advise rather than listen.

The needs of the bereaved are emotional, practical and social, in the long term some will be met by the family or by peer groups such as *Cruse*, but the person left will have to work through most of their problems alone. In the period following the death of a patient the nurse must recognize the needs of those left to grieve and in the absence of anyone else must make herself available to counsel and bring what comfort she can.

Bereavement is the most devastating experience we have to face. It breaks up the established pattern of life and nothing is ever quite the same again. There is numbness, shock, sadness, depression, some guilt, some anger and a feeling of loss that is natural to any acute grief. There will be pining, searching, fear, insecurity, lack of interest and loss of incentive. There will be loneliness and isolation. Such feelings should be expressed freely and not denied. The nurse must listen and her interjections should be directed towards helping the person express their feelings. There is a wide range of books covering the stages of bereavement and the behaviour that accompanies each. These the nurse should read carefully in order to be ready for this very demanding work. It takes a lot longer for a relative to recover after a patient's death than is often realized. It is often two years before a widow can resume an independent and fairly satisfactory life without distress. That this period is important is shown by the number of bereaved spouses that die or develop physical and emotional symptoms within the first year of bereavement.

The nurse should be ready with advice about coping with the many tasks that follow the death of a relative: finding an undertaker, registering the death, notifying certain people, coping with business affairs such as salaries, pensions and insurances. In some families the room and the belongings of the deceased are kept where they were, the whole environment appearing rather like a memorial. In others the clothes are sorted and sent away immediately as though to expunge the person from the memory. It is often necessary to counsel delay as decisions taken where there is a sense of urgency in early bereavement are often taken without due thought, sometimes because of pressure from others who want everything sorted out and put in what is apparently good order, but it is not appropriate or necessary for the nurse to involve herself in advising the relative on the detail of his or her future pattern of life.

The bereaved can be very isolated from their friends. People who were previously friendly become embarrassed. They are vague in offering social help, giving such unwelcoming invitations as 'You must come and see me sometime'. Widows find they are invited out less frequently when they are alone. An infrequent but planned visit from the nurse can help the person work through a plan for coping with the enforced loneliness. However it is seldom that the nursing staff can carry many bereaved relatives in her caseload without penalizing the sick who have first call on her time.

ELDERLY PATIENTS

It is difficult to define old age and identify a group of patients who are elderly. However those over seventy-five and those who are as much as twenty years younger but who have mental infirmity are likely to be particularly dependent upon the health and social services.

Certain changes that accompany ageing should be recognized by the district nurse when visiting so that their effect can be reduced, and that treatable conditions are not attributed to the ageing process and consequently ignored.

In health as well as in disease people's eyesight changes. Often the older person forgets how time passes between each eye test. Some patients need to be encouraged to use the ophthalmic services, so that lenses may be changed if necessary and eye disease detected and treated. Loss of hearing may cause a person to lose interest in people around him whose conversation he can no longer follow, and make him introspective and suspicious. Either condition should, if present in a patient, be recognized by the nurse and appropriate action taken. Smell and taste may be less acute in older people. Some have few teeth or badly fitting dentures. Treatment by a dentist and the provision of new dentures may do much to improve a patient's general health, appearance and well-being.

Muscles weaken and deteriorate with ageing but the process in voluntary muscles can be retarded by exercise and use. Blood vessels lose their elasticity and become rigid, the blood supply to the brain is diminished giving rise to falls and confusion. Joints move less readily and posture becomes increasingly important. There is a tendency for the spine to sag, the head to poke forward, and the hips and knees to be kept bent. This faulty posture combined with increasing physical fraility, and sometimes with giddiness, increases the risk of falls very considerably.

Ageing people find increasing difficulty in remembering facts although they can recall in detail the experiences of earlier years. They retain the ability to think and to reason but do this more slowly. An old person may answer a question several minutes after it has been asked, frequently when the questioner has forgotten about it and is thinking about something else.

Old people need company but they also need to get away from people as they tire quickly. Emotionally they suffer unhappiness as acutely as younger people but their ability to express it is not as good. Unhappiness is often due to loneliness, boredom, social deprivation, loss of work, money and status. Depression accompanies many physical and emotional conditions. It should wherever possible be recognized and treated. Signs of depression include:

1. Personal hygiene neglected. The patient takes an inadequate diet and fluid intake, sometimes even becoming incontinent.
2. Patients experience persistent feelings of sadness and misery.
3. They may become confused.
4. They suffer from sleeplessness.
5. Their physical reactions and thought processes become very much more retarded than is normal for them.

Acute illness is not easy to detect in the older person, illness starts insidiously and changes are not noticed until it is well-established. The temperature may remain subnormal, symptoms may be non-specific. Signs to watch for are: changes in the colour of the face and lips, changes in the pulse rate and volume, loss of appetite, listlessness, incoherent speech, drowsiness, confusion and unexpected incontinence.

It is important that the first signs of confusion in old people are not written off as senility and regarded as irreversable. Early diagnosis and treatment may prevent it becoming a chronic state. Many confusional episodes have an underlying physical condition. It is particularly helpful to consult with a relative of an elderly person who has varying periods of lucidity and whose concentration is minimal. They will know whether the patient normally behaves in this way, whether it can be attributed to some past experience or whether it is a new feature.

When called to a disturbed patient, district nurses may feel extremely vulnerable if they have to decide whether in any particular case the disturbance is such that the patient is a danger to himself or others in the house and how, if this is the case, they can maintain a sufficient measure of support to all involved until the community psychiatric nurse or the social worker arrives to help.

Hypothermia

Slight hypothermia is not an uncommon condition. Some of the important physical signs to be watched for are:

1. Reduced body temperature, body temperature in the elderly is easily disturbed and the sensation of temperature change is blunted.
2. The patient may be pale, the face appear swollen and the skin feel cold.
3. The pulse rate is slow.
4. The respiration rate is slow.
5. There is no shivering reflex.
6. The patient may be drowsy and very slow to react.
7. The urinary output may be increased.

The lower the temperature the more severe the symptoms. All but the mildest hypothermia should be treated in hospital. Reheating the body may cause the blood vessels to dilate and the resultant fall in blood pressure may be fatal.

There are a few important principles that apply when caring for old people. Like everyone else, they need other people to give them a sense of identity and to maintain their self respect. They should be treated with dignity. They should never have anything done for them that they could do for themselves. Care-givers should avoid, as far as is possible, keeping old people in bed. The elderly need to be kept safe, to be kept warm and comfortably clad with sensible footwear.

THE ISOLATED PATIENT

There are various factors that contribute to the isolation of patients from the community around them. Some people are loners, they live alone without being lonely, while others are isolated by such circumstances as bereavement and unresolved grief, or by poverty and they are lonely. Some people are without friends in the area and are therefore alone. Some are isolated because they are awkward personalities.

Society isolates those it cannot easily tolerate, such as the mentally ill, the person who is eccentric and unpredictable, and those who are unclean in person and habits. Certain groups of patients regularly get themselves rejected even by professional care-givers. They are:

1. The uncooperative
2. The poorly motivated
3. The emotionally dependent
4. The manipulators
5. The alcoholics
6. The depressed and suicidal
7. Those with intractable anti-social behaviour

To these patients the nurse has a special responsibility and must be especially objective in her assessment of need, as it is easy to convince oneself that the patient can manage alone when no pleasure is felt in visiting him. Her particular responsibilities for all isolated patients include:

1. The physical care and safety of the patient between visits.
2. Co-operation with other agencies, encouraging other workers from both statutory and voluntary agencies to provide an integrated visiting service, avoiding the situation where they all call on the patient on the same day.
3. Achieving, wherever possible, a balance between bringing people in to offer a service and taking the patient out, e.g. some patients should be encouraged to go back to hospital for the removal of sutures and to revisit the ward, where immediate post-operative transfer to the general practitioner or nurse would mean days and possibly weeks at home alone.
4. Encouraging even a minimal interest in and involvement with the surrounding community.

It is necessary to understand why the lonely patient does not seek to meet others. He may find meeting other people threatening, he may have a low self-image or an unresolved identity problem. Some hostile patients fear their own aggression, some fear reality. In some isolation is at first welcomed, but with the passage of time it becomes so habitual that patients fear to change. Some isolated patients have populated their world with fantasy friends, some relate only to friends and family now dead. Some develop phantom relationships with radio and television personalities to replace real interests. They have often lost the social skills they once had. Sometimes they can be helped to express the good qualities in their friends and neighbours, to sympathize with and encourage others, learning not to be exacting with those who try to help and try to be overtly grateful.

From these small beginnings they may be able to enjoy those professionals they must meet and reach out to any family member or neighbour who would be prepared to try again to establish a relationship with them. Re-education of a patient who has lost his social skills may be possible if he can attend a luncheon club or day centre, rather than have health and social services delivered to him at home. It is not easy for lonely or isolated people to make the effort to approach others. The district nurse may be the one acceptable visitor in the patient's home, and there is a tendency for both nurse and patient who have had to work together on their relationship to feel that they have done enough. However, if the principle of care is to achieve as much independence as possible, another relationship must if possible be established, and in time substituted for that enjoyed with the nurse. The sole purpose for a nursing visit should not be companionship, retraining in social skills should always be attempted.

MAINTAINING STANDARDS OF CARE

Any breach in the duty of care by a nurse to a patient constitutes negligence, but any nurse who performs her duties conscientiously is unlikely to be taken to court accused of negligence. However, although no one is expected to be infallable, with the increasing flow of new knowledge from the universities, research centres and hospitals, practices based on yesterday's knowledge may be negligent. Professional people are expected to know their own limitations. They should question any order or prescription about which they have doubts. If a nurse carries out an order given by a doctor or a senior nurse and harm results, she will not be held negligent unless she ought to have realized that the order was wrong. When a doctor prescribes a drug it is usually taken for granted that the responsibility for the dosage is his. However, when a standard drug is used, if the nurse is given an instruction which strikes her as unusual or unlikely she should query it before carrying out his instructions. If the doctor persists then usually the nurse will not be held negligent if she then carries out the procedure but if she knows, whatever the doctor says to the contrary, that his orders are wrong she is not justified in carrying out those orders. Orders taken from another nurse who is authorized to give such an order are valid but in the event of a nurse being asked to do something she does not feel to be right she has a duty in law to question not only the order but whether the other person is qualified or authorized to give such an order.

The nurse has a duty to maintain the standard of care she gives at all times. No harm should befall a patient because he is receiving treatment. Therefore equipment should be in good order and properly sterilized or disinfected according to the circumstances in which it is used. Sterilization is achieved by autoclaving, and presterilized articles are sealed in packs until use. Disinfection in the home, whether by washing with soap or detergent, boiling in water for five minutes, or using chemical disinfectants is still common. If used without care any method loses its effectiveness, and chemical disinfectants once diluted with water deteriorate, so any solution should be prepared and used on the same day. The recommended disinfectant must be used, some have only a limited range of activity and kill only a few bacteria, and the right strength must be used. A measured amount is essential, a guess unsafe. Articles must be submerged in the solution long enough for disinfection to take place and care must be taken that the solution is not inactivated by such materials as hard water, soap, blood, pus or urine, cotton, nylon, wood or plastic. The chief danger of a chemical disinfectant is not that it fails to kill all microbes, but that those surviving may grow in it very rapidly.

District nurses should pay particular attention to the condition of their scissors, questioning whether they are cleaned thoroughly often enough considering the many different tasks they are used for.

The disposal of syringes, needles and soiled dressings should be undertaken with care. Refuse collectors have complained about handling medical waste packed in paper bags, as there is the risk a dustman may get pricked by a discarded needle in the course of his work. If the needle has been thrown away together with soiled dressing and various swabs used in the surgery it may well be contaminated and dangerous.[7]

Patients often go to great trouble to be ready for the nurse's visit, sometimes making unnecessary sacrifices so to do. An elderly couple kept water boiling on an electric stove throughout the morning to avoid keeping the nurse waiting, but this was at the expense of their heating. It was the nurse's responsibility to see that the practice was discontinued — in this instance a fixed appointment saved the couple money and the nurse time.

It is not easy to identify situations in which people are hurt by thoughtless speech, careless handling or loss of dignity, but when they are it can do great harm to the relationship between nurse and patient and inhibit both in their work together. It is easy to disregard the messages that patients are trying to give and to assume falsely that you can 'cheer people up' who are facing what is to them a great problem, or comfort the anxious with a casual remark such as 'do not worry'. If the problem is real to the patient he will worry and feel depressed unless he can be helped to understand what is happening and accept that something can and is being done, or more problematically accept that nothing can be done. The careless assumption that the patient is grateful for the help he receives from friends or relatives may put him at a disadvantage if he wanted to talk about the problems of dependency. He may recognize the need for help, and know what the relatives must give up in order to give it to him, but he may hate the situation and not care overmuch for the relatives. The nurse can by a hasty action deny him the opportunity to share his feelings with her, when she is the one person who is not directly involved and who should be able to listen and to understand.

Nursing knowledge is a complex combination of behavioural, social and physical insights. It is important that each nurse keeps the balance in her professional reading, and in her work uses and tests stringently theories from all the relevant sciences.

The nurse has a responsibility to keep her knowledge up to date. She should take every opportunity to go to any conferences or discussions which are available. She should read the nursing press regularly and such publications as are relevant to her work. Every district nurse should continue to develop the skills of reading critically, working in libraries, and using indexes that are taught during training. Additionally it is an advantage if she can also acquire the ability to utilize small intervals of study time. As a student, the blocks of time set aside for private study are usually over half an hour. The district nurse who can utilize ten minutes in the surgery once or twice a week not vaguely scanning the journals but purposefully seeking ideas will soon develop the habit. When integrating theoretical insights into practice becomes second nature, a new dimension of nursing practice opens up, skills are enhanced and interest increased.

Post-qualifying courses, multidisciplinary workshops and research projects are some of the formal ways of extending and developing knowledge. Every practitioner should engage in some systematic study every five years in order to meet with others in argument and debate, and have a time away from the job in order to question established procedures and review their standards of work.

THE MANAGEMENT OF CHANGE

Change is constantly taking place in nursing, sometimes its pace is slow but at times it is rapid and bewildering. Changes in practice result from:

1. The introduction of new knowledge.
2. Changes in medical technology which enable patients who hitherto were confined in hospital to be cared for at home.
3. Changes in the administrative structure and in the resources that are made available to the nurse.

Few people like change. It produces stress and releases fears and frustrations, but for the institution it brings new challenges and vitality and banishes complacency. Team leaders in district nursing and their managers have to reconcile two opposing facts in times of change. They have to adapt and use the opportunities available, yet preserve an atmosphere of stability and continuity for both staff and patients. Reconciliation is not always possible, particularly if old established practices are threatened. Change must be anticipated and planned for whenever possible. Consultation makes change more acceptable. It is seen as less threatening when all understand what is involved and those affected by change have had a hand in shaping it. Planned change which can be seen to affect all in the team, and which it is hoped will not involve loss of status but bring benefit to all who participate will generally be acceptable. However there are still going to be some people who resist any change.

Consider the problems experienced by nurses in giving up procedures learned many years before. Some senior colleagues will still rub pressure areas with soap and water despite evidence that it never does much good and in some cases causes harm. Or the response to a change in the rota system for weekend duties. Probably the first question asked is always 'how will it affect me'. In order to manage the psychological resistance to change it is necessary to understand people and what motivates them. It is the individual's notion as to what constitutes his best interest that is important. These interests are not exclusive financial or selfish, nor are most people difficult just for the sake of so being. If the team leader can support the individual's concept of what is to his own advantage, persuasion may be sufficient to carry the reluctant worker into new ways of working.

Some of the most bewildering changes can result from new emphasis being placed on old concepts. It is easy to disregard a new process that is not very dissimilar to one already in practice. When the nursing process was first introduced practitioners tended to say this is what we have always done. Yet those same nurses three years later would hardly recognize the history taking or care planning as belonging to the same service that was previously thought to be adequate.

In times of administrative change, resources are diverted from one aspect of work to another, sometimes with little evidence that good will result. This is extremely disturbing to all members of staff. When change is inevitable there is a right way and a wrong way to implement it. It must be done with understanding. If it has to be drastic and is not negotiable, warning should be given in time for people to anticipate the consequences.

Any change takes time. When a change has been implemented and it doesn't seem to be working immediately the manager and team leader should resist the temptation to change back to the old way. Pressure to do this is strong, and it is often strongest just before there has been time to collect evidence on which to judge the new system. To give up too soon is to waste a lot of time and effort and in some cases financial resources. Real evidence of failure is the only thing that should persuade a leader in nursing to abandon change which in her view would benefit the patients, or the quality of the service given to them.

Implicit in all this is the need for a continual programme of research and interprofessional communication. A research awareness among the practitioners of district nursing will ensure that practice can be tested regularly, revised and re-evaluated when necessary, and its quality sustained. The communication of research findings from practitioner to practitioner and between fieldworker and manager is essential in the field of nursing where most nurses still take their professional decisions alone in the homes of their patients. While reorganization of fieldwork has brought both medical and nursing support to the local centres of district nursing it is still a relatively lonely job. The principles that determine the actions of any particular worker are seldom discussed, as they are often felt intuitively rather than known as a result of systematic study.

The duty of the nurse is to question what she does in order to further her growth as a practitioner of nursing, and enhance her contribution to the work of the primary health care team. She is also an informed member of the public and is often called upon to express an opinion. This puts upon her the responsibility to keep abreast with what is new, to accept that things are always changing, and that she must continue learning from qualification to retirement.

REFERENCES

1. KRATZ, C.R. (1978). The Nursing Care of the Long Term Sick in the Community Edinburgh: Churchill Livingstone.
2. References taken from Hockey, L. Drugs, Danger, Disposal. *District Nursing*, November 1963.
3. The Dangerous Drugs Regulations, 1953.
4. The Home Office publication DD101. *The duties of doctors and dentists under the dangerous drug act and regulations, 1956.*
5. Recommendations made by the Ministry of Health (1953) in response to a request made by the Queen's Institute of District Nursing.
6. WILKES, E. The Effect of the Knowledge of Diagnosis in Terminal Illness. *Nursing Times*, 29 September. 1977.
7. *Disposal of Awkward Household Wastes* (1974). London: HMSO.

FURTHER READING

MANAGEMENT

BROWN, W. (1970). *Exploration in Management*. London: Pelican Books.
FALK, R. (1966). *The Business of Management*. London: Pelican Original.
JACKA, S.M. & GRIFFITHS, D.C. (1976). *Treatment Room Nursing*. London: Blackwell Scientific Publications.
McINTOSH, J.B., 'Decision Making on the District', *Nursing Times*, 19.7.79. Occasional Papers, 75, No. 19.
TINKHAM, C.W. and VOORHIES, E.F. (1977). *Community Health Nursing Evolution and Progress*. New York: Appleton Century Crofts.

THE CARE OF CHILD PATIENTS

BURTON, Lindy, Ed. (1974). *Care of the Child Facing Death*. London: Routledge & Kegan Paul.
BURTON, Lindy, (1975). *The Family Life of Sick Children*, A Study of Families Coping with Chronic Childhood Disease. London: Routledge & Kegan Paul.
HARRISON, Sheila, (1977). *Families in Stress*, A Study of the Long Term Medical Treatment of Children and Parental Stress. London: Royal College of Nursing.
SAUNDERS, C. (1969). 'The Management of Fatal Illness in Children', *Proceedings of the Royal Society of Medicine*, 62, No. 6.

CANCER AND TERMINAL ILLNESS

BURNS, I., & MEYRICK, R.L., (1977). *Understanding Cancer*, A Guide for the Caring Professions. London: HMSO.
CARTWRIGHT, A., HOCKEY, L. & ANDERSON, J.L. (1973). *Life Before Death*. London: Routledge, & Kegan Paul.
Terminal Cancer at Home, (1965). *Lancet*, 1–799.
HILTON, J. (1967). *Dying*. London: Pelican Books.
SAUNDERS, C. (1978). *The Treatment of Intractable Pain in Terminal Cancer*. London: Edward Arnold.
WILKES, E., 'The Effects of the Knowledge of Diagnosis in Terminal Illness, *Nursing Times*, 29th September 1977.

BEREAVEMENT

GORER, G. (1965). *Death, Grief and Mourning in Contemporary Britain*. London: Cresset.
KUBLER–ROSS, E. (1976). *On Death — Dying*. London: Tavistock Publications.
LEWIS, C.S. (1961). *A Grief Observed*. London: Faber.
MARRIS, P. (1958). *Widows and Their Families*. London: Routledge & Kegan Paul.
PARKES, C.M. (1975). *Bereavement*, Studies of Grief in Adult Life. London: Penguin Books.
SPECK, P. (1978). Loss and Grief in Medicine. London: Baillière Tindall.
YOUNG, M., BENJAMIN, B., & WALLIS, C. 'The Mortality of Widowers', *Lancet* 1963, 2, p. 454.

THE ELDERLY

AGATE, J. (1973). *Geriatrics for Nurses and Social Workers*. London: William Heinemann.
BROMLEY, D.B. (1974). *The Psychology of Human Ageing*. London: Pelican.
BROMLEY, D.B., 'Speculations in Social and Environmental Gerontology', *Nursing Times*, Occasional Paper, 21st April 1977.
CONI, N., DAVISON, W., & WEBSTER, S. (1977). *Lecture Notes on Geriatrics*. London: Blackwell Scientific Publications.
HAZEL, K. (1960). *Social and Medical Problems in the Elderly*. London: Hutchinson.
KEMP, R. (1965). *A New Look at Geriatrics*. London: Pitman Medical.
STORRS, A.M.F. (1980). *Geriatric Nursing*. London: Baillière Tindall.

THE ISOLATED AND THE DEPRESSED

Dominian. J. (1969). *Marital Breakdown*. Harmondsworth: Penguin.
PRIESTLY, P., McGUIRE, J., PLEGG, D., HEMSLEY, V. & WELHAM, D. (1978) *Social Skills and Personal Problem Solving*. A Handbook of Methods. London: Tavistock Publications.
ROSS, Mitchell, *Depression*. London: Pelican Mind Special.
SNELL, H. (1977) *Mental Disorder*. An Introductory Textbook for Nurses. London: George Allen & Unwin.

RESEARCH

MACLEOD CLARK, J., & HOCKEY, L. (1979) *Research for Nursing. A Guidebook for the Enquiring Nurse*. London: HM & M Publications.

CHAPTER 4

The Promotion of Mobility and Independence

Immobility brings problems to all systems of the body and dependency robs the individual of dignity. Therefore the principal object in domiciliary nursing is to achieve as much mobility and independence for each patient as possible. There are many factors that influence recovery, the targets set for any patient depend not only upon the severity of the disability but also on the emotional and psychological disturbances that accompany it. The degree to which any remobilization programme succeeds, however, depends upon his persistent hard work and the enthusiasm and commitment of all who care for him. The patient's own temperament is important. Those who are determined to overcome their disability and have the tenacity of purpose needed to fight back to independence have a head start on those who give up easily or those who find dependency more comfortable than the continual striving to help themselves. While all patients are damaged by frustration and repeated failure, most can be encouraged to persist despite setbacks if their nursing plan is based upon an accurate assessment of their particular strengths and limitations. The nurse must learn to recognize how every patient copes with his problems and what physical, emotional and intellectual skills he is able to draw upon.

THE CONCEPT OF REHABILITATION

Rehabilitation is the concept used to encompass all the activities undertaken by statutory and voluntary workers who are helping the patient struggle to regain independence. Rehabilitation nursing is the special responsibility of the nurse to help such patients learn to move in as coordinated a way as possible, to do as much as they can for themselves, and accept responsibility for those decisions they make together. Rehabilitation is frequently an inappropriate word as the process is not reserved for patients who are going to get better, the same principles apply even when the prognosis is poor. Much district nursing is concerned with maintaining whatever movement and independence is left to the patient rather than improving his performance. Patients should be helped to be as independent as possible until just before death. No one should remain absolutely still, even if the patient is unconscious his limbs should be moved regularly and positioned properly.

There are three models of rehabilitation applicable to domiciliary practice. Each is helpful, none entirely satisfactory. The first is simply that rehabilitation starts with good, basic nursing care which is modified gradually as the patient is able to take over the care for himself. This is satisfactory providing that the basic concept of nursing care is wide enough to include the changes in behaviour caused by the patient's disease processes and his dependency, together with an awareness of the burden of care put upon his family. It should also include the social consequences of the illness within both the household and the neighbourhood. The second model is based on the assumption that health is an ideal state in which the physical, emotional, intellectual and spiritual elements are in balance. In practice such a state of health is very difficult to define and for the majority of patients it is unattainable however skilled the care they receive. A more realistic model describes health as a utility and rehabilitation as a relearning of basic physical functions such as continence, washing, dressing, standing and walking. This too can be limiting, but if it is taken together with the idealism of the second model it can lead to a systematic relearning or replacing of the capacities lost through illness.

Apart from the different models that are adopted there are different styles of rehabilitation nursing in practice. In some cases a routine is prescribed for the patient who is urged to accept the imposed discipline. In others when the plan is drawn up the patient is asked to cooperate and his suggestions are incorporated into it provided they do not profoundly change the original scheme. Both styles are sometimes appropriate but should be regarded as temporary stages in the transfer of responsibility back to the patient and his family. The third style is the most difficult to initiate but generally results in the most successful programme. It involves the patient and his family planning the programme from the start or as soon thereafter as possible. At each visit the nurse enters into a dialogue with them as to the best way to progress. The patient's consent for any change in the plan or any new activity is essential, and indeed it is desirable that whenever possible the patient himself suggests and initiates activities that he would like to follow.

TEAMWORK IN PLANNING CARE

As the patient becomes aware of what help he needs the nurse uses her experience of how others have coped to suggest ways of overcoming his problems. She can anticipate the rate of progress and where difficulties may arise, she brings to the home not only her own professional skills but also the resources of allied services in the community. Medicine, nursing, social work, physiotherapy and occupational therapy are the professions most closely involved in planning rehabilitation programmes, but physiotherapists and occupational therapists are seldom employed in sufficient numbers in the community to visit all patients who need them.

The district nurse must therefore acquire the ability to stimulate patients to make the necessary efforts to regain mobility and independence and the skill to plan a programme of activities that will keep his muscles flexible and his joint movements precise. She must be able to persuade the patient and his family to reorganize their environment in such a way that the patient has room to move around while still retaining stable furniture to hold on to for safety. All this will be in addition to her basic nursing care and health teaching. This is planned to ameliorate those factors that may have contributed to the onset of the disease, and those inhibiting recovery and return to normal life.

It is not possible to teach the exercise routines that might be followed by particular patients except individually or in a class by experienced district nurses and physiotherapists who will subsequently act as consultants and advisers to the nursing team. Supervised practice is essential as faulty methods involve risks to the patients and to those who nurse them Since independence involves coping with everyday activities the occupational therapist may suggest modifications that could be made in the home, they can recommend for the patient new skills often supplemented with mechanical or electrically driven apparatus. The social worker will work with the patient building up his self-esteem, counselling him and encouraging him to fight those limitations that can be overcome, and helping him come to terms with what cannot be changed.

All professional help is limited, and in any social service department there are a variety of workers with different levels of skill. It is important that the nurse knows whether she is working with a professionally qualified colleague or one with narrower technical competences, and what help each can bring to the situation. If for example a patient, following amputation of his leg, is unable to reconcile himself to his disability, the nurse may contact the social services department for help. Should she put undue emphasis on his physical condition the person who visits may be a technician to measure the patient for crutches or a wheel chair, rather than a social workers skilled in helping the patient through an emotional crisis.

GAINING THE PATIENT'S COOPERATION

It is in the patient's best interest that from the onset the nurse assumes that he will regain at least some independence. As shown in Chapter 2, her skill lies in assessing what is reasonable to expect him to achieve, and estimating the amount of cooperation the patient and his family are able and willing to give her. At the first visit she will look for clues to the activities that mean most to the patient, those for which he would be prepared to make and sustain considerable effort in order to be able to do again. It is important that the patient chooses those activities which are important to him and are attainable within a reasonable time. The doctor or the nurse may suggest the first small tasks to be relearned but the patient must agree wholeheartedly, and see them as part of a progress towards something he wants to do. Later because of the high regard he has for those helping him he may agree to attempt more than he first thought possible, to learn different skills from those he had used formerly, but first he must want to make the effort and be interested in the possibility of achievement.

Some people who have had special skills will not be able to face doing badly what they once did well. A patient after a stroke may never again play his piano, but he may be able to take an interest in the musical education of his grandson, or learn to listen more critically to music on the radio.

THE SUPERVISION OF RELATIVES' WELLBEING

The patient's relatives, friends and neighbours provide the bedrock on which any rehabilitation programme is built. Despite the pessimism of some social commentators they shop, provide meals, check there is clean linen and visit in the evenings to see all is well. Relatives and neighbours need teaching, by demonstration and detailed explanation, not only how to care for the patient, but how to encourage and support him through difficult periods. They should also be encouraged to talk about the way in which they cope with the extra work involved and how much it interferes with their own activities. Some may be helped by just talking about their feelings and their relationships with the patient and others in the household.

Caring is hard work and patient's relatives need health supervision too. They often have a full-time job, or are managing a growing family. Anxiety and fatigue can inhibit their appetites, leading to a diet of snacks. Infection either already in the house or brought by a visitor is initially more dangerous to the harrassed care-giver than to the patient, although the latter will be subjected to it in a more concentrated form if the care-giver succumbs. There is stress in all caring and district nurses should always be alert to signs of stress in the family. The relative whose behaviour patterns change, or whose responses appear inappropriate give cause for concern. Relatives and friends always feel guilty if the patient gets worse, more breakdowns are associated with the patient's deterioration than with overwork, and when they feel guilty they keep at bay the people who are most likely to understand their problems and be able to help.

When stress appears to be excessive, the nurse should:

1. Seek an opportunity to have a private talk with the patient to find out what he thinks about the situation.

2. Seek medical advice both in relation to the relative's health and the patient's wellbeing should the care-giver no longer be able to cope.

3. Check all the dangerous drugs in the house.

4. Arrange for company, support and help from other relatives, friends, voluntary organizations or statutory services.

5. Make realistic contingency plans in case there is a breakdown in the arrangements to ensure that the patient has someone to call on in case of emergency.

When a patient becomes severely disabled there may be distress and tension within the marriage. The nurse should be alert to the sexual deprivation experienced by patients and their relatives. Normal intercourse may be difficult, painful or even impossible to achieve and without informed counselling the marriage may break down. Even when alternative ways of love-making exist it causes unnecessary distress when patients are not properly instructed in the most appropriate method they could use. Some forms of contraception are impossible or impractical. Patients with deformed hands and upper limbs may not be able to introduce caps or vaginal contraceptive devices. Intrauterine devices may lead to menorrhagia and are difficult to insert into patients with serious hip malfunction. The pill carries various side effects and is not always suitable. Often patients hesitate to ask about such matters and nurses and doctors attending patients with disabling conditions should always enquire directly whether they need help and if necessary seek marriage guidance or family planning advice as appropriate.

Illness does not affect a patient in isolation. The inter-relationships of all members are altered and may become strained. The team members who visit the home have a responsibility for the integrity of the whole family. Breakdown may be averted by prompt relief. The provision of help in the home, marriage guidance, day hospital care, holiday admission or assisted holidays may ease the burden enough for all the family to work out their problems together. It is seldom satisfactory to try and find solutions for each person singly and in a piecemeal manner. Only a joint approach to the crisis will enable the family to continue to function as a unit.

THE ASSESSMENT OF NEED

There are three levels of need to be assessed in order to plan a programme of work with a patient:

1. Needs that the patient can or soon will be able to meet unaided.
2. Needs the patient can meet with limited assistance or those he can be taught to meet.
3. Needs the patient cannot be expected to meet himself even in the long term.

The goals that are set for the patient in the first instance are those in the first category so that as soon as possible the patient and his family see that there is something they can do and some old skills they can recover. The second group needs more time, often more courage on the part of the patient and more commitment from those caring for him. To meet these needs the patient must be fully involved in planning his programme of care, and be able and willing to accept the responsibility for his own part in it.

PLANNING NURSING CARE

There are three stages in any rehabilitation nursing plan:

1. The provision of good basic care in the initial stages, having regard for the physiological disfunction resulting from the disease process.
2. Achieving as much balance and coordination as possible between

the affected and unaffected parts of the body. This is most easily demonstrated in the case of a hemeplegic patient when the balance is a physical one, but it can also be an intellectual balance when a patient with multiple sclerosis is encouraged to use his planning and organizational skills in order to minimize the amount of actual physical help he needs.

3. Achieving as much independent movement as possible together with the re-establishment of interests outside the immediate environment, and activities that involve intellectual as well as physical effort.

The programme may start with the patient able only to make the effort to grip a sponge, but this is an essential preliminary to washing his hands himself. In the case of a bronchitic patient it may be taking deeper breaths and later controlling expiration. The nurse in the meantime will be taking the initiative in all matters of care including: correcting his posture, supervising his diet and fluid intake, combatting incontinence or constipation, ensuring that he can communicate his needs to others, and in an emergency can get help quickly.

The nurse will involve friends and family but she must impress upon them that those things the patient may and can do, he should do. She should also make clear that the patient's routine will change constantly as his condition fluctuates. His need for help will vary from day to day according to his physical or emotional strength and buoyancy. It is difficult for relatives to learn when to help and when to refrain from helping, particularly if the patient gets cantankerous and sometimes abusive when he is disappointed in himself. It is much easier to do things for a patient than to help him do things for himself, and well-meaning relatives can render a patient dependent if they cannot stand by him while he struggles.

During the initial period the nurse will seek to remedy any conditions which impede progress towards mobility. The following guidelines relate to the most common conditions that can undermine the patient's capacity to help himself or render him permanently dependent.

CONDITIONS WHICH MUST BE IMPROVED BEFORE REMOBILIZATION IS PRACTICAL AND OTHERS WHICH IMPEDE RECOVERY

In the long-term care of patients at home several conditions cause extreme discomfort and tend to occupy the patient's thoughts to the exclusion of all else. They include constipation, incontinence, decubitus ulcers and oral ulceration. Others like dehydration, malnutrition and weakness due to inactivity are less painful but must be reversed before any remobilization programme is started.

DEHYDRATION

Dehydration may result from insufficient intake of fluid or excessive loss. The signs are:

1. The skin is wrinkled, having lost its elasticity it remains in a fold if it is pinched.
2. The patient is dull and lethargic.
3. The tongue is dry and leathery in appearance.
4. Thirst may or may not be present. Older people often have a diminished sense of thirst.
5. The urine is scanty in quantity and concentrated.

When dehydration is suspected the cooperation of family and friends is necessary as a strict regime of drinks every hour or two must be organized. Rehydration is essential before remobilization is started as the patient's cooperation is unlikely to be forthcoming until his fluid balance is corrected and he regains vitality.

MALNUTRITION

Poor health and depression may have reduced the patient's appetite as well as making it difficult to shop for food or cook it once it is puchased.

Vitamin deficiency

The diet may be short of vitamin C, and this will delay healing, predispose to pressure sores and make the patient tired and apathetic. Lack of vitamin D contributes to a high incidence of fractures, particularly in housebound people. Health teaching has, however, to take into account the fact that overdosage of vitamin D can cause high blood calcium which may result in kidney and brain damage. Iron deficiency anaemia is common, probably caused by a shortage of iron in the diet, but it may also be due to small internal haemorrhages. Patients on a prolonged course of diuretics may suffer shortages of minerals such as potassium and magnesium as well as some vitamins. Protein intake can be markedly reduced particularly in the elderly. If a simple but detailed nursing plan is worked out with the patient the excitement of a new routine, together with the encouragement and personal interest of the nurse, will generally stimulate the patient to eat more.

Obesity

In the elderly particularly this is a very difficult problem. While fat people are at risk of heart disease, diabetes and arthritis, they are also much more difficult to nurse and impose a great strain on those who care for them. As an immobile patient probably only requires about 800 calories to maintain his weight, reduction of diet in a chairbound patient sufficient to promote a weight loss has to be so severe that there is risk of vitamin and mineral deficiency. It is very important, therefore, for members of the primary health care team to take very seriously the health teaching of all people on their lists who are more than 13 kg overweight.

INACTIVITY

Activity is the key to continued health, ageing organs quickly lose their function and efficiency if not used. When physical activity declines, muscles and joints lose their powers, simple tasks become difficult and painful, and well-meaning friends recommend rest. In consequence the patient becomes increasingly immobile. It is necessary to point out that exercise and movement are helpful and that the term *exercise* includes simple household tasks, walking, washing and dressing. Precise tasks like combing their own hair, fastening buttons or rising from a chair are useful achievements by which progress can be measured. Inactivity can lead to gross deformity of joints and to contractures. It also predisposes the patient to disease in any of the systems that rely on muscular activity, such as the circulatory, respiratory or digestive systems.

ORAL ULCERATION

Whenever a patient complains about a sore mouth it should be taken seriously. While some ulcers are the manifestations of serious underlying disease and require expert diagnosis and treatment, even the insigificant and wholly innocent ulcers which people get in their mouths are very distressing. Ulcers sometimes make it impossible to wear dentures and often the soreness alone will prevent patients from eating a proper diet. When examining the patient's mouth in a poor light it is not easy to see oral ulceration nor to see their extent and distribution which is an important factor when assessing the probable cause.

Jagged teeth or dentures can cause traumatic ulcers in the mouth. Their distribution is discrete and if the biting habits of the patient are observed these can usually be detected quickly. They should heal within ten days of removing the cause.

Patients who suffer from ulcers in their mouths frequently overtreat them with proprietary preparations. They may not cure the ulcer and in some cases may make the surrounding tissue soft and sore, causing the ulcer to spread. Thrush may infect the mouth in the elderly sick. Infective mouth ulcers may be due to Herpetic or Vincent's infection in which case there is a risk to young children in the family. The equipment used for the patient's mouth toilet must be kept separate and care must be taken over the disposal of waste water and swabs.

Internal diseases such as the anaemias give rise to sore tongues. Painful ulcers on a red shiny tongue are characteristic of iron deficiency anaemia. The patient with pernicious anaemia complains of a burning tongue but it does not generally ulcerate.

Necrotic ulcers together with exhaustion and slight jaundice are indicative of agranula cytosis, leukaemia or ulcerative colitis.

Neoplasic ulcers are often greyish with an irregular border. Sometimes a plaque like lesion appears on the lower lip, or the lateral margin of the tongue. They may also be found on the floor of the mouth, the gums and the inner surface of the cheeks.

THE CARE OF THE MOUTH AND TEETH

The care of the mouth has four aims:

1. Maintenance of comfort
2. Cleanliness
3. Keeping the mouth surfaces moist
4. Preventing infection

The health of the mouth depends upon an adequate flow of saliva which is stimulated by:

1. Adequate fluid intake — if the body is short of water all secretion becomes more viscid. The elderly and some patients having drug therapy lose their sense of thirst and are then very much at risk of oral ulceration.
2. Mastication
3. Psychological stimulation

Illness diminishes all these factors, so attention must be paid to encouraging the patient to eat proper meals and have frequent drinks wherever possible. It is also useful to give attention to the way his food is served. Even if the patient has meals-on-wheels delivered they can be made to look attractive on the plate by making fresh gravy or sprinkling fresh parsley over fish. This can stimulate the appetite and cause an anticipatory saliva flow. Lemon juice is a salivary stimulant but it will lose its effectiveness in a short time if over used.

Two other factors that cause soreness of the mouth are: mouth breathing which allows evaporation from the tongue, and the presence of a thick mucus coating on lips, tongue and teeth.

Wherever possible the patient who needs dental treatment should receive it. Apart from urging the patient to drink and to chew, the mouth must be kept clean and if necessary the mucus should be removed with bicarbonate of soda but this is not pleasant and should be used sparingly. The lips can be moistened with petroleum jelly or liquid paraffin. The use of an antiseptic mouthwash sometimes brings comfort but its effects are very short-lived.

The patient who is able to clean his own teeth with a brush or scrub his dentures is unlikely to get an infected mouth. When the patient is not able to manage, the nurse or relative must undertake mouth cleansing. It is sometimes convenient to use swabs, but as an alternative a baby's toothbrush is useful as it is soft, not too uncomfortable, and it effectively removes the debris left after meals.

Some patients, such as those with leukaemia, suffer from bleeding gums and for them treatment must be exceedingly gentle. All blood clots should be removed, but care should be taken to avoid starting the bleeding again.

Patients with anaemia who have a brown, dry tongue, with a distressing smell and taste may be helped by having pure glycerine applied to the tongue.

When undertaking mouth care it is important to maintain the patient's self respect. It is undignified to have to submit to having one's mouth swabbed and teeth cleaned. No patient should ever be left without their dentures for long without a good reason.

PRESSURE SORES

Pressure sores are painful areas of dead skin and underlying tissues, sometimes called decubitus ulcers. The only real treatment is prevention. Tissue submitted to pressure frequently or continually will be damaged. Skin is more resistant to pressure than either fat or muscle so that when the skin turns red some damage to internal tissues may have already occurred. There are two types of pressure. The first is produced by direct compression force. It will present itself insidiously and the damage may not be noticed for several days. The second is the shearing force which is produced when the weight of the body runs parallel to the source of pressure. The latter is often the cause when the patient at home drags himself or is dragged up the bed in the absence of care-givers who have been taught how to lift. There are several factors in the environment that may increase the effect of the pressure such as wetness, irritants such as urine, soap or other chemicals that cause allergic reactions. When the skin surface is broken bacterial action will exacerbate the damage caused by the pressure.

Certain patients have conditions that predispose them to pressure sores. They are the acutely ill, the patient whose diet is deficient in protein or in vitamin C, those whose oxygen supply is impaired through vascular disease, accident, anaemia or large doses of steroids, patients with metabolic disorders.

The patient who cannot move is in extreme danger. Pain, drugs, paralysis and extreme age are among the conditions that render a patient immobile. A patient in pain may not risk moving but the administration of drugs to remove the pain may make him drowsy and still more reluctant to move. Patients are seriously at risk when the pressure is unrelieved because they are semi-comatosed. Oedema is also a predisposing cause of sacral sores.

The elderly patient's skin is particularly vulnerable to pressure because the outer layer of skin is thinner and less well supplied with sebaceous secretion. There is a shortage of water in the tissues and subcutaneous fat is often reduced. Also in this age group healing powers are diminished and medicaments applied to the skin are less effective as absorbtion through the skin is reduced. Drugs injected too shallowly are an additional hazard that may damage tissues and result in pressure sores.

Sometimes patients at home gather together their treasured possessions and unconsciously damage themselves on hard objects secreted in their beds or chairs. Rings, watches, a rosary with a large crucifix, a tin box of photographs, can all exert pressure if the patient sleeps on them.

The prevention of pressure sores includes general as well as local measures. Any malnutrition should be treated and any protein or vitamin deficiency reversed. The patient should have an increased fluid intake, particularly if he is elderly, as the increase of protein may raise the blood urea. Any anaemia should be treated. The patient's doctor should be persuaded to prescribe analgesics rather than sedatives. Locally the area over which the weight is distributed should be increased, ripple mattresses may be needed to do this and to reduce the time any particular tissue is under pressure. Sheepskins are comfortable to lie or sit upon. The patient can be taught to move just sufficiently to reduce the pressure on his buttocks or elsewhere but he must be very self disciplined and make these movements regularly every few minutes through the day.

The skin must be kept clean and dry. Massage may increase the circulation momentarily, but if the skin is red or damage to the underlying tissue is suspected it may do harm. Relief of pressure is the only effective answer.

The treatment of pressure sores includes: persuading the patient to take a diet high in calories and in such proteins as meat, fish, eggs, milk. Some patients find the fortified milk drinks useful in supplementing their diets. All should drink at least two litres daily. The slough should be removed from the ulcer, and any factors that prevent healing such as infection, oedema, defective oxygen supply, and impaired nerve supply should be treated or modified as far as possible.

CONSTIPATION

The word constipation is not easy to define. Its meanings include infrequent and sluggish action of the bowel as well as difficult defaecation and the passage of hard, dry, faecal material.

The most frequent causes of constipation are:

1. That the sensation produced when the mass of faeces passes through the sigmoid colon into the rectum is ignored.
2. That there is a lack of roughage or dietary fibre in the diet.
3. Due to a lack of exercise.
4. Due to emotional factors such as excitement or fear.

Constipation may be secondary to a range of conditions, including:

1. Such psychiatric states as depression or chronic psychosis.
2. Disturbance or disease of the colon. The slow transit of the contents of the colon from ileum to caecum may be hastened by the increase of dietary fibres in the diet. The colon may be constricted by diseases such as carcinoma, diverticulitis, haemorrhoids and fissures.
3. Such other diseases as myxoedema, diabetes, spinal cord injuries, and any paralysing condition such as a stroke may be accompanied by constipation.
4. Diuretic drugs, antidepressive drugs and misused laxatives all can cause constipation.

The side effects of constipation are distressing and often the patient is too ashamed of them to seek help. They include: soiling, incontinence, nausea, flatulence, abdominal pain and anal soreness.

The principal treatments are:

1. Peristaltic stimulants such as Senna or Dulcolax.
2. Bulking agents such as bran or cellulose preparations.
3. Stool softeners — Drochyl Sodium Sulphosuccinate.
4. Evacuants such as glycerine suppositories and enemas.

There are dangers in using saline aperients, castor oil and liquid paraffin, the first two affecting the electrolyle balance and the latter the absorbtion of vitamins.

Constipation in the elderly patient is more persistent and less easily treated. In these patients the passage of faecal matter through the colon is slower, a decreasing physical activity diminishes also the rhythmic contractions of the colon which are dependent upon posture and muscle tone. Sensation is also diminished, including the awareness of the need for defaecation and the rectum is often only partially emptied at any one time. Many elderly patients suffer from constipation frequently in an advanced stage. It is accompanied by pain, vomiting and dysphagia. A patient may be found to have thrush in his mouth and throat which will mean he cannot even drink without pain and becomes dehydrated. The diet of the elderly patient is often inadequate and the easy and convenient foods they take lack the roughage, the protein, and the fluid needed to promote regular bowel habits. There are three dangers of constipation in elderly patients at home:

1. Faecal impaction may occur.
2. They may become toxic if the colonic content is stationary too long.
3. They may strain excessively in order to pass a hard, impacted stool and die of heart failure.

Enemas are frequently the method used initially to relieve severe constipation. Once the bowel is emptied the patient should be followed up within four hours if possible, and at least within twelve hours, not only to observe the immediate effect of the enema but to start health teaching. This also should be followed up in order to reinforce the instructions given and try to prevent the condition recurring.

INCONTINENCE

Incontinence is not uncommon. It is a very distressing condition which may result from any incident involving a loss of consciousness or of one's voluntary control of defaecation and urination. Incontinence, defined in the Oxford dictionary as wanting in self-restraint, is a very negative word implying failure to attain or retain a skill usually achieved in childhood.

In childhood it used to be sufficient if a child was in control of his sphincter muscles in time to go to school, but now with many mothers at work and many children at nursery school or play group, pressures are exerted to reduce laundry and become continent earlier in life. Enuresis is regarded as a shameful disease whereas formerly it was accepted as a temporary condition that would be outgrown. In middle age some women are incontinent as a result of trauma in childbirth. It may also follow unskilled or careless catheterization, as well as damage to the spinal cord or degenerative disease. In old age the proportion of people who are incontinent may be as high as 25–30% of all over 65 years.

Faecal incontinence is often the result of faecal impaction. The bowel should be completely emptied; two or three enemas are often needed. The daily sanitary routine should then be re-established through drug therapy and corrected diet.

Incontinence however minor, whether urinary or faecal, should be investigated.

SPURIOUS INCONTINENCE

Lack of mobility may cause incontinence. The stiff joints of a patient with arthritis may prevent him getting out of a low chair, or out of bed, in time to get to the lavatory. Once accidental incontinence causes a lonely person to give up trying to maintain their standards of personal hygiene they will deteriorate. Regular visits to the lavatory are important for all patients, particularly if they are elderly. Cold houses and draughty lavatories do not encourage the regular emptying of the bladder and the bowel that can prevent the onset and the prolongation of a period of incontinence. In some cases it will be enough to provide a walking frame or rails and raising the lavatory seat may help, but if this is not enough a commode or a urinal may be loaned to the patient.

The nurse is often in the best position to make the preliminary observations needed for the accurate diagnosis of incontinence. She should report on the nature of the incontinence, its frequency when it occurs and how the patient reacts to it. All patients have some emotional response to an episode of incontinence and this should be borne in mind when making care plans. There are three approaches to the management of incontinent patients in most cases the nursing plan will reflect all three in varying proportions.

1. *Prevention*

This will include making the patient as mobile as possible, increasing his sensory stimuli by changing his position, giving him something to look at, to do, or to listen to. The nurse must also ensure that his bowel and bladder are emptied regularly.

2. *Protection*

The patient's clothes, furnishings and bedding can be ruined by incontinence. They should be protected. His skin should be cared for by keeping it dry and clean and, if necessary, protected by barrier cream against wetness.

3. *Retraining*

This should start with an attempt to re-establish control of bowel and bladder. The patient should be taught how to use and manage any appliances that are provided. In addition the nurse should counsel the patient and his family who have a very disagreeable condition to cope with and who need continual support throughout each episode. An optimistic attitude is important if they are to make realistic plans to retain the patient's dignity and help him regain his independence.

Catheterization is generally recommended in cases of long term illness, terminal illness or continual urinary incontinence. However it is not always the method of choice in the elderly confused or intermittently incontinent patient.

Certain guidelines on management may help the patient's family, they include:

1. If a patient is made to feel dependent he may cease to make any effort for himself, become incontinent and be very difficult indeed to retrain.

2. The care-givers need to recognize and avoid feeling resentful when they care for the patient. The patient himself may become quite aggressive when he is incontinent. The patient has to learn with the help of his relatives, friends and nurses to manage not only the physical but also the emotional aspects of this condition.

3. A patient who is left alone without anything to do or to be interested in is more likely to suffer from incontinence than one who is made to feel part of the family or community.

4. Untreated depression will lead progressively to decline in self-respect, to self-reproach, guilt and even more depression.

5. Regression in behaviour, the reasons for which may lie in childhood relationships, may be reinforced by the wrong attitudes demonstrated by the nurse or other care-givers. Scolding or chiding the patient or treating him as a child not only destroys his self-respect and dignity but it can trigger off a childlike response which impedes retraining.

Other aspects of home management include the coordination of services for the household. The health visitor, occupational therapist and social worker may be helpful. Alterations in the home may make access to the lavatory easier, and equipment such as a commode, chemical closet and special chairs can be obtained. There should be a supply of incontinence pads and other disposable garments; a special laundry service will relieve the family of some washing. If the nurse has access to the surgical appliance workshop she may find a technician with imagination who can help her find appliances and suitable apparatus for the special needs of her long-term patients. Any plan that might reduce the distress of incontinence should be considered.

The problem of disposal of soiled material is not inconsiderable. The plastic bags for collection of incontinence pads get very offensive within a few days. They must be carefully sealed between use, not be overfilled as they can get very heavy, and they should be kept in a well-ventilated space where the surrounding area can be washed and kept clean. Deodorant sprays and wicks do not solve the problem but they do help.

The Information Service of the Disabled Living Foundation answers enquiries relating to the problems of incontinence apart from medical matters and issues information on equipment, clothing, services available and sources of financial help. Individual enquiries can be made in confidence to the Incontinence Adviser, Disabled Living Foundation, 346 Kensington High Street, London W14 8WS. Telephone 01–602–2491.

STARTING A REMOBILIZATION PROGRAMME

All programmes should involve relatives and friends who can encourage the patient. Exercises need to be performed regularly throughout the day, not just when the nurse visits. Certain patients will work very hard once they realize that they have the choice of speeding or retarding their own recovery, and this re-establishes their self-respect. Others need constant urging, they need friends and relatives to remind them of what they should do as well as to watch with them for signs of improvement.

The programme should be simple. Many people, especially the

elderly, get anxious if they think they have forgotten an instruction or got it wrong. If necessary the nurse should write down what the patient is to do. Initially this should not exceed two or three tasks at the most. It is important for the nurse to give realistic expectations at each stage. She should start with something within the patient's capacity so that there is the satisfaction of achievement with little effort involved. The movements should be increased gradually, becoming more difficult and more varied only when the simple movements are mastered. For example, a patient with osteoarthritis of the knee will commence with a leg-lifting exercise as he sits in his chair, lifting his leg as far as possible ten times every two hours. He will then graduate to holding each lift for a count of five, before letting his leg down. The holding time can be increased to six and later to ten so that the patient is not only exercising his joint but also measuring his improvement. If it is considered suitable to continue movement against resistance a shopping bag can be hung over the ankle and items such as packets of tea, sugar or flour used as weights.

Since independence involves coping with every day life it is necessary to get the patient out of bed, sitting, standing and walking if possible, with as short an interval in bed as possible. The older the patient the more debility follows bedrest and only when complete rest is specifically prescribed should the patient not be encouraged to move all his joints regularly and lift each part of his body off the bed or chair at least once an hour.

THE SPECIFIC NEEDS OF PATIENTS PARALYSED BY A STROKE

Anger and anxiety stimulate the sympathetic nervous system and may be associated with a rise in blood pressure. Emotional tensions often complicate the lives of hypertensive arteriosclerotic patients. The patient's personality makeup, therefore, may include attributes which predisposed or precipitated the stroke. Certainly the same characteristics will influence his reaction to his illness and the manner in which he will attempt to solve his problems. In this respect he will be helped or hindered by the attitudes of his family and friends as well as those of doctors and nurses.

The major factors that will influence the course and outcome of the disease are as follows:

1. The family support and encouragement.
2. The motivation of the patient.
3. The disabilities left by the stroke such as:
   (a) the degree of brain damage

(b) defects in sensory and coordinating function

(c) the amount of paralysis and the loss of dexterity

(d) speech disorders such as dysarthria and aphasia

4. Undesirable attitudes on the part of the patient which may include rebellion and aggression, an unwillingness to conform to medical or nursing routines and treatments. The patient may become spiteful to those who would help him, or he may use his disability as an excuse for avoiding responsibility.

The first need of the patient is for good nursing. As Strickland says, 'there is always the danger of pressure sores developing on the affected side as the patient will tend to roll over onto the paralysed limbs'.[1] He should sit up during the day and each night be placed firmly on the unaffected side when he prepares for sleep. The patient's paralysed arm will become permanently damaged if it is not exercised regularly and positioned correctly.

The patient should be helped to move each joint from shoulder to fingertips every hour. It is important that full extension of the shoulder is attempted twice a day. The good hand can be used to steady and support the affected hand in as many activities as possible, for example: washing his face, cleaning his teeth, taking cool drinks and eating. When not exercising the affected limb should rest in a natural position, the hand and wrist supported. The palm facing upward, and the fingers outstretched. Footdrop is another hazard that can be prevented. The foot and ankle should be moved regularly. Excess weight taken on a borrowed or improvised cradle in the bed, and a firm support inserted to keep the foot on the affected side at right angles to the leg.

The patient should use his good arm as he feeds himself, washes, moves about the bed as well as when he reaches out for his radio, a drink of water or fruit juice which should be on a table at the side of the bed nearest the unaffected limb. This causes the patient to lean towards the stronger side and corrects the tendency to bend towards the paralysed side.

The first movement that the patient is taught may have to be rolling over in bed. The patient must be sufficiently near the side of the bed to be able to hold the mattress or the arm of a steady chair. The movement is started by turning the head and shoulders towards the affected side, the sound leg is crossed over the affected leg, the sound arm crosses the body and holds the mattress. The patient pulls with his arm and rotates his hips, simultaneously turning onto his affected side, his sound knee and thigh act as a brake. Rolling back towards the strong side requires greater effort. The strong foot is inserted between the weak ankle and the bed and the affected leg is hitched over the strong one. The sound hand takes the affected hand outwards and upwards towards the affected side. A twisting movement of the hips together with a swing of both arms will enable the patient to roll onto his sound side with a little help.

The patient once having managed the rolling quickly learns to take his weight on the sound elbow and lift first his head and shoulders and then continuing the movement gets into the sitting position. The supporting arm must be positioned far enough away from the body to provide support without straining the shoulder. The patient, as soon as he sits up in bed, can be encouraged to sit with his legs over the side of the bed. These movements are both described and illustrated in the booklet 'Training for Independence.'[2]

Once the patient can sit on the bed supported by his good hand he and the nurse can practice a balancing exercise. She rocks him gently backwards, forewards and sidewards. He must resist the rocking and then maintain his balance in the sitting position for a minute or two, once or twice a day.

If the doctor agrees, most patients should be sitting out of bed for bedmaking from the second or third day. Each day the period out of bed should be extended until he is sitting up for long periods. Chairs, bed and commode should all be the correct height, that is when the patient is sitting his foot should be flat on the floor and the knee bent at right angles.

When the patient is ready to be transferred from the bed to the chair or commode, the nurse must be ready to support him, propping him up with her body, preventing him from falling towards his weak side. She must stand on the affected side holding his upper arm with her forward hand and supporting his back with her other arm. He is encouraged to stand upright on his strong leg, when he is steady he moves his hand to the far arm of his chair and the nurse eases him into the chair. The nurse controls the affected leg by placing her foot in front of the patient's foot to stop it slipping and she presses her leg against his knee to keep it straight until it is safe for him to sit down.

The return to bed is easier. The chair is moved so that when the patient stands he can place his strong hand on the bed to take his weight as he sits on the side. He can then shuffle up the bed and be helped if necessary to swing his legs in, once he is in the correct position in bed. It is easier if the pillows are removed from the bed until the patient is back and then put into position.

Meanwhile the patient should move all the joints of the upper limb regularly ready to learn to dress and undress himself.

Within a few days a walking aid should be procured and adjusted so that the handles just reach the patient's wrist. His first walk should be to the lavatory. The nurse should stand by the affected side and a relative should follow with a chair in case the patient cannot manage the whole journey without rest. In due course most patients will change the Zimmer for the tripod or for a walking stick. Ninety per cent of all patients, it has been estimated, walk again after a stroke.

The patient who has suffered a stroke may need the help of a speech therapist to diagnose the type of speech disorder and to prescribe treatment. Where this is so the therapist should be brought into the team as soon as possible in order to participate in the assessment and the total care plans. The patient needs treatment from the start in order to get maximum benefit from it and the relatives need support and teaching if they are to carry on her work. Speech therapists are not always available for patients at home. In such cases the nurse might find the following guidelines useful.

The aphasic patient may not have any difficulty understanding what is said to him or what is said about him by careless friends and relatives. The patient may only have difficulty with articulated speech or he may have problems finding words or forming sentences.

Language is an acquired skill, the meaning and associations of words are stored in the brain, and the ability to use them depends upon recall through the integrated functioning of the nervous system. The patient who, although unable to read aloud, can recognize written words can communicate his needs either by using printed cards or, if he is able, writing on a pad himself. Use of the written word depends upon his dexterity and is affected by his basic education and his familiarity with writing. Some patients after a stroke may be unable to interpret the words spoken to them, in these circumstances the written word is not likely to be useful either. Sign language may be used but only sparingly as it may deter the patients from struggling to regain speech.

Anxiety often complicates the re-establishment of communication when the patient suffers from a speech disorder, and his difficulties are increased if he does not wear his dentures, his hearing aid or his glasses. The nurse must speak slowly and quietly on an adult level. She should talk to him as though he understands even though he may not. She should never talk of him in his presence as though he were not there. Friends and relatives should spend as much time as possible listening to his attempt to speak and trying to understand what he says. Gestures and pictures may help. A book of pictures, phrases and words may be compiled to act as a reference book when verbal communication is too exhausting.

If brain damage interferes with reception, the nurse or relative should speak clearly and slowly. They should face the patient all the time, avoiding any background sounds which might distract the patient or distort the sound of their voices.

If the patient has problems with interpretation, only a few people should visit him at the same time. They should use only a few familiar words, express only a few ideas and these only one at a time.

The first communication that should be established either verbally or non-verbally is a call sign, that can be used in an emergency. Patient and family can then evolve a series of calls, distinguishing between the urgent and not so urgent. Special calls indicating the need to go to the lavatory, loss of balance, or when the patient gets into an uncomfortable position are useful. As in the long term a few specific signals help to make caring simpler they help also to reduce the stress experienced by the relatives.

Sometimes the patient's life is made miserable by the fear of choking. He may then resist having anything to drink and run the risk of dehydration and/or urinary infection. The patients who are most inclined to choke are those who have lost the power of coherent speech, therefore, the nurse and family must interpret and anticipate the needs he cannot voice, and for such a patient a special 'choking signal' is essential so that he can get help immediately.

REHABILITATION FOLLOWING AN OSTOMY

The patient who returns home with a stoma may make an uneventful recovery. He may however be a very sick man if his underlying condition is not operable, or a very miserable man if he is not able to adjust to his body's disfigurement. He and his family may take a very gloomy view of such a radical alteration in the way he excretes faeces and expects others to withdraw from him in disgust. He may have only partial control or not completely reliable control over his excretions and expect never to be able to go out to public gatherings again. This is a particularly gloomy view but it still persists in many communities. The stoma, however, is only one of his problems and his rehabilitation must be planned around the prognosis of the underlying condition. A patient whose ulcerative colitis has been cured by colostomy is generally better able to return to a normal life than the patient with malignant disease, although his stoma may be more difficult to manage. The first essential is sympathetic understanding of the anxiety and distress that patients and their familes may suffer. The second is efficient collection of the drainage. The process of rehabilitation is shared between hospital and community and depends upon good teamwork. It includes counselling the patient about the operation as soon as it is suggested giving the patient and his family the opportunity to voice their fears and ask their questions of the doctors who are responsible for the diagnosis and the recommended course of action.

It is common practice in most hospitals to arrange for the patient to meet another who has had such an operation and to put them in touch with the appropriate voluntary organization. This may be the Colostomy Welfare Group, the Ileostomy Association or the Urinary Conduit Group.

Post-operative care in hospital is one of the most positive influences in rehabilitation. If the patient is given confidence that his stoma is manageable, he will quickly learn to manage it himself. All patients need practice in using their equipment before returning home. Some general instructions about management and diet, and guidance on the disposal of used bags and soiled dressings should also be given.

The patient should have written down for him the name of the appliance he is using, its size and type, so that he can hand this to his general practitioner when he needs further supplies. There are a number of stoma clinics in hospital outpatients departments with a qualified nurse who is trained and experienced in the management of stoma. This permits easy access for the patient who needs expert help from time to time. Home visiting by a stoma nurse is also available in some areas.

Problems such as a persistently irregular and unpredictable bowel action, irritant adhesives, and excoriation of the skin occur in a minority of patients. The district nurse should consult first with her hospital colleagues about alternative management but sometimes the answer comes from experienced domiciliary colleagues, the voluntary associations and the appliance suppliers, all of whom have met the problems before.

The district nurse has problems when the hospital service is not fully developed and she does not have the necessary updating on appliance and new techniques of patient management. The nursing management will know if there is a stoma care nurse consultant locally and be able to put staff in touch with her. If the patient's appliance is causing trouble all manufacturers have fitters who will advise the nursing staff. They will send samples and literature to both patients and professional staff and often mount film shows and conferences to bring up to date those who are likely to be recommending their product.

The problems patients do have are often complicated by loneliness. When he is supported by a caring family and has friends around him most difficulties can be overcome. When the appearance of the stoma is the cause of distress to the patient he may feel mutilated, and think that others will be revolted. He may withdraw from friends and neighbours, fearing their rejection. The attitude of the nurse is important, she must understand and accept that he has these feelings, but she must also accept the stoma and urge the patient to do so in order to live as normal a life as possible. She must be able to teach him about diet, grooming and exercise as well as the management of the stoma and the care of the appliances. He is entitled to exemption from prescription charges and the nurse should be able to help him apply for this and any other benefit to which he is entitled.

THE REHABILITATION OF THE ELDERLY

In the elderly a disability may occur suddenly or develop insidiously until incapacity brings the problem to the notice of the primary health care team. In both cases improvement may be slow, laborious and expensive in terms of both time and energy, if the results are going to be sustained. Early mobilization is essential; enforced rest causes physical changes and apathy diminishes motivation. Incontinence, muscle weakness and joint stiffness are some of the consequences of immobility in the elderly.

The progression from bed to chair should only be the first step towards remobilization as venous stasis and venous thrombosis complicate chair rest in the same way as they occur in the bedfast patient. It is important to ensure that old people can rise from their chairs. They should be able to stand in a stable position even when their weight bears more heavily on one side than another. The chair should not be so deep that the patient cannot put his feet on the floor. The chair back should be vertical so that the patient can swing his trunk forward at the same time as he exerts pressure from the arms of the chair with his arms and extends his hips and knees. The height of the chair depends not only on the height of the patient but also upon the flexibility of his hips. Chair arms should be stout enough to support the patient even when he is straightening up.

If the patient is well enough to be up he should be encouraged to dress. To be comfortably and simply dressed is more dignified than sitting around in bedclothes, and it is generally warmer. The act of dressing moreover provides purposeful activity for the patient that can be increased as skill develops. Well fitting shoes are necessary for all patients, particularly those with defective gait.

The elderly patient needs to practise balancing exercise. If the bed has a headboard or a footboard that is stable a board may be placed in front of the bed legs. The patient is then seated so that his well shod feet are against the board. Using the end of the bed he can then draw himself out of his chair into the standing position. This exercise repeated frequently can do much to restore his balance. Once standing the patient can transfer his weight from one foot to another and alternate feet can be raised off the floor as a preliminary to walking. Once the patient is able to stand he should learn to walk, using an aid rather than relying upon another person, so that he relies on his own balance. It is essential however that the aid is the right height, too high a 'pulpit' type aid will throw the patient backward, a walking stick that is too long will cause the patient to fall to the opposite side. All walking aids held in the hand should be long enough to reach the styloid process of the ulnar so that the patient can walk with a straight arm.

While the patient is still in bed he will have started to regain independence by learning how to feed himself, to wash and to dress. When he is ambulant his first journey will be to the lavatory and the bathroom. His next target should be to gain competence in the kitchen, in walking in the garden preferably where he can see and speak to other people.

It is rare for the disabled elderly to do too much but very easy for them to do too little. It is quicker and easier for the nurse or the patient's family to do something for the patient, rather than to encourage them to do for themselves.

EXAMPLES OF REMOBILIZATION

One of the most exciting rehabilitation programmes was that devised by a student district nurse for a patient who, following a slight stroke, had become obese and constipated. Her colon was impacted, she had diarrhoea, her flat was filthy, she had no visitors and she lived on a diet of carbohydrate and fat. The nurse was called by the milkman because the home was so offensive. Over a period of two months the student emptied and re-educated the patient's colon. She reorganized her diet. She persuaded a home help to come and help her get the patient and her home clean. She acquired a commode and a wheelchair and taught the patient how to move from one to the other. Within six months the patient, who had once been a good cook, was able to get out to her kitchen and prepare her own food again. She was unmarried and had no close family, however a nephew and his wife were contacted and agreed to visit her. It was a great triumph for the patient to be able to bake a cake for them. They never knew how near to despair she had been and she was able to entertain them graciously enough for them to want to visit her again later in the year.

Another case of imaginative rehabilitation was seen in the home of a patient severely crippled with rheumatoid arthritis. She was a very private person who chose to live alone. The nurse together with the hospital appliance officer and a local carpenter planned handrails and ramps to make a walkway between the patient's bedroom, bathroom, and a table on which she had an electric kettle and a toaster. Her diet although supplemented by meals-on-wheels was very monotonous, her struggle to keep her person clean was painful and protracted, but the joy of staying in her own flat outweighed all the inconvenience and discomfort she suffered.

THE COST OF DISABILITY

When a patient is disabled life becomes increasingly expensive. No small savings are possible when the housewife cannot shop around for the most satisfactory purchases, when she cannot buy in large amounts or carry heavy bulky parcels even short distances, and paid help is costly. Alterations to the home are often necessary to maintain independent functioning, and heating costs are high. Some symptoms create their own expenses. The patient who is clumsy and slightly incontinent as the result of multiple sclerosis may spend several times as much on clothes and shoes as her healthy neighbours. She will damage furniture, have more breakages, spend more entertaining her friends to meals out, or travelling by taxi to visit them. The greater her struggle to live a 'normal' life the more she will need to spend.

There is constant strain when one person is dependent upon another. The service given is seldom adequate. It is not always given in the manner the patient would choose or at the most convenient time. Many disabled people are, to a limited extent at least, dependent upon friends and family, and in most cases dependency involves some financial obligation. There is a strain put upon those caring too. In the family of a patient who had a stroke five years ago the husband had got up every day at 5.30 a.m. to prepare a meal and care for his wife. He left for work at 7.30 a.m.

and returned at 6 p.m. to start the housework. Caring may cause education and training to be interrupted, career prospects diminished and this may mean a limited earning capacity.

Housing is often inadequate and unsuitable when there is need to house special transport. More room is needed in families who support a handicapped person in order to give the young people in the household privacy and when the patient needs constant attendance the care-giver needs a room adjacent to the sick room.

Despite the increase in institutional care for the disabled there is not enough for the short-term stays that are not booked ahead. Therefore the families who meet a sudden crisis and need relief have to be desperate before emergency admission can be procured and families are thus denied the spontaneous recreation that most households take for granted.

Despite the emphasis on self-help the scarcity of rehabilitation specialists still means some patients never get all the help they need. There are unfortunately too many occasions in which the communications between home, hospital, health centres and surgery are not as good as they should be. There is still inadequate follow-up of patients once their active care is finished in hospital; neither is there a consistent pattern of supervision following home care.

THE ATTITUDES OF SOCIETY TO THE DISABLED

Disabled people embarrass those who are inexperienced in caring. When someone is confronted with a patient they occasionally ignore them and talk to other people as though the patient was both deaf and dumb. This undermines his dignity. The inexperienced nurse too may fail to see each patient as a unique individual. This is her barely conscious defence against the depression and pain experienced by the patient and his family. She may then too readily identify them with the group of patients who share the same diagnosis and disability.

Some people assume that the welfare state provides adequately for the handicapped and disabled. Some able-bodied people go so far as to infer that they are living at the expense of the rest of the community. The disabled themselves tend to feel that this is the majority opinion and that with some exceptions they live in a rather uncaring and critical world. It is necessary, therefore, that the task of remobilizing a patient and the promotion of independence is undertaken with understanding and compassion, in order that the persistent urging needed to promote activity is seen as caring and not as nagging, and supervision or health teaching is not thought of as less than *real* nursing.

REFERENCES

1. STRICKLAND, E. How can you help. Nursing Times Community Outlook 'Stroke', *Nursing Times*, November 1978.
2. Queen's Institute of District Nursing. (1970) *Nursing in the Community*. London: The Queen's Nursing Institute.

FURTHER READING

AGATE, J. (1973). *Geriatrics for nurses and social workers*. London: William Heinemann.

BROCKLEHURST, J.C. (1973). *Textbook of Geriatric Medicine and Gerontology*. Edinburgh: Churchill and Livingstone.

DARDIER, E.L. (1980). *The Early Stroke Patient: Positioning and Movement*. London: Baillière Tindall.

DOBSON, P. (1974). *Management of Incontinence in the home: A Survey*. London: Disabled Living Foundation.

HAZEL, K. (1960). *Social and Medical Problems in the Elderly*. London: Hutchinson.

KRATZ, C. (1978). Nursing the Long Term Sick in the Community. Edinburgh: Churchill Livingstone.

MANDELSTAM, D.A. The Active Management of Urinary Incontinence. *Modern Geriatrics*. **4**, pages 507–512. December 1974.

MANDELSTAM, D.A. (1977). *Incontinence — a guide to the understanding and management of a very common complaint*. London: Disabled Living Foundation.

NORTON, D. (1970). *By Accident or design*. London: Churchill Livingstone.

Nursing Mirror. Incontinence Nursing in the Community. *Nursing Mirror*, **144**. 14th April 1977.

Nursing Times. Physiotherapy Helps Nursing. *Nursing Times*. 1962.

The Queen's Nursing Institute. (1970). *Nursing in the Community*. London: The Queen's Nursing Institute.

ROBERTS, I. (1977) *Discharges from Hospital*. Royal College of Nursing Research project, **2**, number 6.

STORRS, A.M.F. (1980) *Geriatric Nursing*, London: Baillière Tindall.

CHAPTER 5

Understanding People

Were you to ask a group of colleagues why they thought people caught colds, their answers would include theories about germs, about resistance to infection when they are tired, hungry or cold, and about how stress and anxiety increase vulnerablility. Each theory has some validity and some people will think one explanation preferable to another. So it is in all aspects of human behaviour. There is no single body of knowledge that will provide a guide to practice, and district nurses need to know about various theories and concepts which may throw light on the problems they meet. Theories of human behaviour are not statements of universal truths, this is a field in which new material from research and clinical practice is constantly being published and in which controversy is rife.

We think we must know about behaviour because we have all many years of life experience, but the surest principle in the study of behaviour is that once a person seeks to understand his thought processes or the forces that induce him to behave in a certain way, distortion sets in. It is more comfortable to think that one's behaviour is rational than admit that we all at times behave in inappropriate ways that are not under our complete control.

Behaviour is influenced by many factors, some physiological, some environmental, much is learned from early experience, some is determined by the expectations of people we wish to please. It is not often possible to prove the theories that are put forward because there are too many variables in any set of circumstances to be able to compare one form of behaviour directly with another. Therefore the evidence that underlies any theory or concept must be examined very critically. A single caseload is a very small sample in which to judge ideas about behaviour and illness but it is all most of us have. A simple test of our own thinking is to compare our ideas with those of others to see whether they are shared at least to some degree. Readings from psychology, social psychology and sociology can provide frameworks against which ideas can be tested, discussing the readings with others, applying the principles to commonly encountered experiences will clarify the concepts and give additional insights into the relationship between health and behaviour. Some of the concepts may also be used to understand the working of a staff group, or to improve the skills of supervision. In this chapter a few concepts are outlined in order to show their relevance to district nursing and to encourage students to seek more detail in the specialist textbooks.

The study of behaviour is important for four main reasons:

1. It helps the nurse to understand the normal growth and development that she will encounter in any family or in any group.

2. It helps her recognize when there is deviation from normal.

3. It helps her anticipate the normal reactions to stress and to plan her work accordingly.

4. It is necessary to understand the management of patients with mental disorder and the support needed by their families.

WHAT IS NORMAL BEHAVIOUR?

It is not easy to define normal behaviour, nor to say how much anyone can deviate from what society thinks is normal without being regarded as abormal. Some behaviour that is at present thought of as abnormal would not have been unusual in earlier times, or in a different cultural setting. Some behaviour may be tolerated in times of stress but be unacceptable in other circumstances. Normality is neither a constant state nor uniform for any individual. It is best described as a process of adapting to the environment.

The ability to estimate the degree of abnormality in any situation comes with experience. The experienced Sister will not confuse the misery of a lonely widow with a frank depression although the signs may be very similar. This has a parallel in physical care where abdominal pain may be a temporary acute indigestion or a symptom of intestinal obstruction.

The nurse may be alerted by a change in the behaviour of a relative under stress, a daughter who had been concerned for her parents may suddenly deny all problems, alternatively agitation may replace indifference. However, confused patterns of thought and bizarre behaviour in a person who had previously appeared methodical and reasonable would be regarded as abnormal. Abnormality can be defined as behaviour that is incongruous in the particular setting, having regard to the individual's usual behaviour as well as his inclination and ability to meet the norms set by society.

There are people whose behaviour is deviant and who will not seek help. They are known to the nurse only because she visits the home. They may include the very anxious, the depressed, those with obsessional or hysterical behaviour patterns and those with social symptoms such as truancy or lying. Their management is often the responsibility of a relative, supported by the nurse until such time as the condition causes undue suffering or is thought to be dangerous and intervention is essential. It is in the anticipatory guidance that can be given and in the containment of rigid and disturbed patterns of behaviour that the nurse fulfils her role as promoter of mental health.

When individuals or a group of people are unable to accept the life style or the beliefs of their culture they are sometimes called deviant. There are always people who will question established practices and challenge the existing systems. Without them there would be no progress, but society as a whole resists change and views those who differ from the majority as troublesome. Deviants are sometimes more compassionate than the host society; they are sometimes more intolerant. The one thing they have in common is that they are different. In some societies deviants are regarded as mad or bad. Those who are thought of as deviant in one generation may be quite acceptable to the next, but while they are deviant they may be vulnerable to illness yet denied the attention given to the conforming. The death and morbidity rates of children born to single parents exceeds that for children born into families with two parents, despite a change in the public attitude to marriage. Homosexuals, alcoholics and drug-takers are among those still regarded as deviant by many in our society.

GROWTH AND DEVELOPMENT

Individual growth, whether physical, mental or emotional, proceeds through stages. The rate at which people pass through each stage will vary but the sequence in most cases will be the same.

In cognitive development Piaget[1] defines four stages from birth to twelve years, when the child develops language, ideas about number, volume and weight and eventually the capacity for abstract thinking. Freud

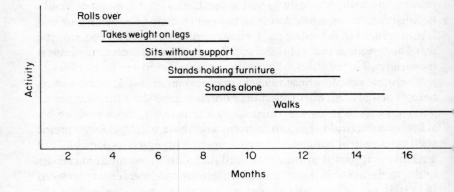

Fig. 3. Some stages in the physical development of a young child, including the range of time in which it normally takes place.

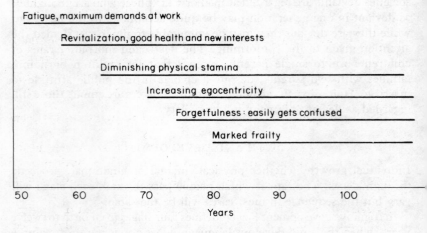

Fig. 4. Some stages in the ageing process.

defined stages in personality development[2] and Erikson[3] subsequently suggested eight stages throughout life in which psychosocial change was taking place. He describes for each stage the relationship between the individual development and the social and cultural context in which it takes place. He indicates who are the significant people that influence growth and what form each development should take. Erikson's chief concept is that of identity which he believes is developed through life but particularly in adolescence when the young person seeks friends of his own age and learns to be himself. This development he follows into late adulthood (which enhances its value for district nurses) where the old person is struggling for integrity against despair, the outcome of this his terms suggest can be either wisdom or renunciation and disengagement from social life.

INDIVIDUAL DIFFERENCES

Each person's genetic structure will determine his physical characteristics and to some extent his intelligence, but as soon as a child is born these inborn factors are modified by his environment. Thomas Chess and Birch[4] list nine characteristics which scored on a three point scale measure differences in children's temperaments as early as two months. They include activity, distractability, response to a new person or object, attention span and the child's intensity of reaction to stimuli.

There are eight groups of factors that influence the way in which people behave.

1. Each person has a different physical makeup resulting from their genes, their life-style including nutrition, their freedom from disease or malfunction. The maturity or otherwise of the nervous system, the hormone circulation, the metabolic rate are some physical systems which have an obvious bearing upon behaviour.

2. Intelligence and the ability to see relevant relationships between objects and ideas.

Everyone has some capacity to learn, this may be stimulated to its fullest capacity in a few but it can also be damaged by birth injury, disease or trauma, inhibited by adverse experiences or distorted by fear and anxiety.

3. Flexibility of thinking is not necessarily a component of intelligence, it is the capacity for imagination and creativity the ability to see alternative ways of coping with difficulty.

4. Experiences: these are unique to each person, because how each interprets their experiences differ, as is what, and how much, they learn from them.

5. The temperament of the individual, their enduring traits that result from their development and their adjustment to circumstances. It includes such dispositions as willingness to take responsibility, to share, vitality or depression as well as the strength of their needs and feelings.

6. Emotional stability which is primarily probably the result of very early experience denotes a person's capacity to make and sustain relationships. To have a consistent view of reality and a realistic appreciation of what they can or cannot do.

7. Beliefs and moral standards are the basis for many conscious decisions as to how one behaves. They can also be the reason for characteristic behaviour, not easily understood by the onlooker.

8. The influence of other people: throughout life there are people who the individual will wish to please, and in so doing he will take on those characteristics which meet the other's expectations of him until the feelings and actions he has adopted become automatic and part of his particular behaviour pattern.

The concept of self and of identity are important in the care of patients. Illness, particularly if prolonged, can alter the person's concept of himself and diminish his sense of his own identity. If, for example, the breadwinner in a family suffers a stroke, he may need to rebuild his self esteem and accept a modification of his sense of identity before he can concentrate on regaining his physical independence.

SOME CONCEPTS FROM PSYCHOLOGY

Originally psychologists described personality in terms of drives and instincts. The basic drives were hunger, thirst, sex, the need to rest when tired, the need for bodily protection, the need to avoid or seek relief from pain. Each drive was associated with an emotion that in turn sparked off specific behaviour. Events too were seen as determining behaviour, thus early deprivation was association with inevitable problems later. Current thinking regards the individual less as a creature of habit at the mercy of his environment, and more as a person capable of striving for self fulfilment.

PERCEPTION

Perception is partly biological, as information is picked up from the surroundings by the sense organs and transmitted to the brain. From these sensations are built up groups of ideas which determine how the individual reacts to his environment. The sense organs cannot attend to all the stimuli bombarding them, neither can the brain cope with all the available material, so in every aspect of perception there is selection of material. What is selected depends upon its relative importance to the person and this in turn is the result of his past experiences.

Trying to understand how people see their environment is important. What they see is for them reality. So for a new patient with diabetes his problems may loom as large as sharks while to the nurse they appear only as tadpoles. It is no use telling him they are only tadpoles, he must be helped to cope with the sharks. It is more difficult to judge how a person perceives himself. Although from time to time certain actions are revealing, the total picture is inevitably distorted by what the observer thinks about the person as she comes to know him better. It is not possible to know what it feels like to be Jonathan with multiple sclerosis. It is possible to understand the characteristic features of the disease, and how people manage in various ways to come to terms with the increasing disability and cope with the fear of dependency. But there is no one in exactly the same position as Jonathan, no one knows what he is thinking, how much he fears the future, what resources he has to cope with the problems and which problems he must deny if he is to avoid despair.

When people misperceive they may not have selected enough stimuli or they may have selected the wrong stimuli. When a relative sees herself as inadequate it may be that she attends only to those problems she cannot solve for the patients and the mistakes she makes but not to the comfort she is able to bring. The stimuli may be perceived but misinterpreted. The nurse may be aware that a patient's relative is often out and think that she has to go a long way to the shops but the relative may be escaping from the house during the nurse's visit because she cannot bear to be asked to help with bedmaking and face the evidence of deterioration in the patient's condition.

MOTIVATION

This is the term given to the forces that induce a person to act in a certain way. Both physiologists and psychologists isolate needs which must be met if the person is going to survive satisfactorily. The need for food and oxygen is obvious without either they will die, but in addition each individual has a need for love, and security, for new experiences, as well as for praise and recognition. Maslow's[5] general motivational hierarchy is a range of needs, starting at the bottom with the most essential that must be met first and rising to the demands for personal satisfaction

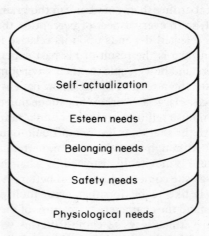

Fig. 5. Maslow's hierarchy of needs.

Maslow distinguishes between the lower motives which are aroused through deficiency and are urgent determinants of behaviour when they are not satisfied, and the higher 'being' motives which come into play when the survival needs and normal social needs have been met. The higher motives are associated with the development of the complete person.

It is very difficult to disentangle one's own motives. Any motive may produce a variety of actions, and any response may be the result of a variety of motives. Moreover there are frequently many motives, not all of them harmonious, that at any one time determine action. The nurse who stops for coffee with a patient during a busy morning may be tired and hungry, the patient may need to talk, the next patient on her list is very demanding, but she may affirm and be quite sincere in her belief that she stays only to support and counsel the patient. It is even more difficult to attribute motives to others and it is rarely possible to anticipate their behaviour on this basis.

Not all motivation is conscious, no one is fully in control of their behaviour all the time, forgotten experiences long past can be a potent force in behaviour. In some circumstances the person's capacity for creative and imaginative responses to new situations is restricted because of their rigid and repetitive patterns of behaviour that once might have served a purpose but are now an automatic reaction to anxiety or fear. Thus the patient whose well-being depends upon his ability to adopt a new daily routine or a radical change of diet may be impeded in his rehabilitation by behaviour that is unexpected and even he can only partly understand it. Relatives are also subject to this phenomenon. A diabetic patient may be subject to stress every time his family has sweets, not because he craves for chocolate or toffee but because his spouse will always offer him one before helping herself and when the box was actually before him saying no was too difficult. Yet the wife cannot break the habit of sharing learned as a child. The patient who needs to be accommodated in a ground floor room may find it unacceptable to upset a little used 'best' room and prefer to remain a virtual prisoner in an upstairs bedroom.

LEARNING THEORIES

Another method of approaching the study of behaviour is to think of all behaviour as a learned response. If then the result of a certain course of action is favourable or well received by people who matter to the individual or who have authority over them it is likely to be repeated, and frequent repetition will make this behaviour habitual. If the response to a certain action is unfavourable or antagonistic the behaviour will be suppressed, and when no response is made the behaviour will in a short time be discontinued. This fairly predictable pattern is basic to the possibility of retraining by means of rewards and punishments. Enuresis and the diseases of addiction are so treated. People do not however only learn what we expect them to learn, consider a child cared for by a deaf grandparent, he cries quietly and is not heard, he screams and is heard. Subsequently he screams immediately he needs attention even when he is not cared for by his grandmother. We teach patients to be demanding when we do not meet their needs properly, withhold information or do not have sufficient respect for their feelings.

THE CONCEPT OF SOCIAL INTERACTION

The concept of social interaction is developed from the assumption that a person develops his identity according to the way in which other people respond to him. No one can develop fully alone. A personal identity exists only when people recognize that identity and treat the person accordingly. The interaction depends upon at least two people having contact with each other, which can be verbal or non-verbal. Its nature will depend upon the perception each has of the other, both as an individual and in their particular role. It follows therefore that any new patient's reception of the district nurse will be conditioned by how he feels about her, what she wears, how she speaks, how he feels that she treats him, what he expects a district nurse will do and whether he has any confidence in the help she will give him. This will determine how easy it is for them to start working together, what form her teaching should take and what goals they should set for his rehabilitation.

The helping relationship is a particular form of interaction in which one person offers to help the other find a satisfactory way of coping with their problems. It depends upon the person in need seeing the possibility of using the help. An agreement to work together is important as help cannot be given without the consent of the person to be helped. This consent must be given freely because ultimately helping must lead to self help if it is going to be sustained. For example, relieving the pressure on a patient's relative with extra home help time when she fears she cannot cope is only a temporary expedient. The fear will return in another guise unless she can talk about it and about the future, what will be expected of her, what help she can expect, and what would happen if she really could not manage. It is important to recognize that the patient must talk this through herself and not just have the answers given to her. Too often helping is thought of only as assistance given and accepted, but it is wrong to think that where there is need help will be welcomed. It is true of course that if the person in need recognizes that certain information or skills would be useful to him he will accept them but only on his terms. In some cases need is not always recognized. Frequently, solutions that are suggested are not acceptable particularly if they involve the person in changing habits or long-held attitudes.

There are dangers in helping too, should the helper not be able to enter into a proper relationship with the other, she may try to compensate by doing too much which can create dependency. She needs accurate medical knowledge in order to set the limits to what the patient can or should do, and an approach that can make her encouragement acceptable. If she cannot and the patient is not able to motivate himself he may be able to hide behind his diagnosis and become a permanent invalid. Helping sometimes fails when either the nurse, patient or relative is afraid to allow negative feelings to be expressed, and consequently problems can never be worked through between them. The patient who has heart failure may have to give up an active life and accept one that is much quieter. This new identity must be sustained by friends and family making him feel of value even though his activities are restricted. Once they have convinced him of his abilities they must help him to do what is safe but stop him taking risks. They will then need the primary care team as much as he does to provide accurate information about what he may or may not do, as well as support and encouragement to talk about their feelings and listen to the patient talking about his until their understanding is mutual.

SOME BEHAVIOUR ENABLES OR PREVENTS ANOTHER FROM ACCEPTING HELP

Because the concept of self is so dependent upon others' responses it is extremely vulnerable. In circumstances when one's self is threatened or one's control over the environment is limited, interaction that in any way diminishes the person in their own eyes or apparently reduces their status as an independent person also reduces the likelihood of them asking for or accepting help. The respondent to a phone call from a would-be suicide must accept the caller without giving any overt signs of agitation, in case this is interpreted as impatience, anger or rejection and the caller takes fright and rings off. Giving help is not simple either, anxiety can make us particularly harsh with people who have problems. A mother may shout at, or call her child silly, when a mishap occurs because *she* is anxious, not because the child could reasonably be expected to anticipate the danger. The district nurse may exasperated with the patient who needs help but 'does not want to be beholden to anyone', or have difficulty accepting the problem family without criticism.

Certain concepts can be identified that help to clarify the process of interaction and the problems that beset both those giving and receiving help.[6]

Ambivalence occurs to some extent in all situations where a choice is made between alternatives. The desire to be slim is in direct competition with our appetite for certain foods. Ambivalance is the situation that occurs when a favourite chocolate is offered to a slimmer, who must then decide whether she wants it more than she wants to slim. Emotions also have two dimensions; one may love another yet in some respects be indifferent to them. Likewise hate or dislike is seldom without a contradictory element. Generally one group of feelings very much outweighs the opposite one, it is when the desire to do something is balanced by a fear of doing it, or a desire not to do it that trouble arises. Thus, although a person may recognize their need for help, they may not find it easy to ask for help since it involves putting themselves in someone else's hands, revealing their inadequacies and disclosing their private affairs.

The patient who has completed his treatment in an intensive care unit will not wish to be reminded of his dependency and may avoid meeting staff after discharge, alternatively he may need to return to demonstrate his independence to them. The patient who shares her despondency about a weakness in his family relationships or failure in marriage on one day, may resent the district nurse at a subsequent visit when he is feeling better and wishes he had not been so outspoken. The need for help is not the only factor and the person's feelings about seeking help may not be consistent. Sometimes the need for help outweighs the need to keep problems hidden, other times the feeling prevails that one should struggle alone.

The helper has also to develop skill in understanding how it feels to need help. This is not sympathy, but a feeling for and with the person in difficulties. The individual who neglects an elderly relative, or the mother of an abused child need help from someone who can recognize what is happening to them and why: feeling sorry for them or liking them is immaterial to this basic feeling for and with them in their plight.

Helping other people is an extremely demanding occupation, it is necessary for staff who counsel others to be able to call on other colleagues for help. This is often provided by management, sometimes by an independent counsellor, but frequently it is another fieldworker with the capacity to listen and understand who helps best.

The responses and the reactions that are common in ordinary social contact have to be modified in a helping relationship. The person needing help is always vulnerable, yet in some cases may present as angry, aggressive, suspicious or hostile, so that the helper feels threatened. The expedience of disarming the person to ward off these emotions is not helpful. Antagonistic emotions directed to the helper may be justified if the latter has been guilty of carelessness, but they may be so directed because they cannot be expressed to anyone else with safety, or the person may always react to anxiety with anger and aggression. Rigid and unrealistic this approach may be but the underlying problems are real enough. The emotions must therefore be accepted in order that the problems may be opened up in discussion as unfaced problems preclude any genuine helping.

UNDERSTANDING HOW GROUPS WORK

The interaction in a helping relationship is usually between two people, but it can occur in a group. The success of such activities as weightwatchers, alcoholics annonymous, or groups of parents of mentally handicapped children are among the best known. The nurse in the community may be involved with groups as a resource person. Types of groups may include patients suffering from sickness or disability, specific groups facing fundamental changes of routine such as diabetics, patients undergoing regular renal dialysis, those who have ileostomies in common, or who are being rehabilitated after strokes or people trying to give up smoking. Nurses also use families as support groups to strengthen the person with the immediate problems be they patient or relative. When the nurse persuades the parents of a patient with a carcenoma of the lung to care for his children and so release his wife to be with him constantly, she is using the group strengths of the family.

When initiating a self-help group the aim is that every member of the group should contribute from their experience and that the group will give to each member information and ideas about their mutual problems, as well as the comfort and encouragement that will enable them to draw on their own untapped resources, find new methods of coping with their problems and have the courage to persevere.

Now each time anyone tries to arrange for people to meet together or uses initiative to help them they put themselves in a special relationship with the group. It is as though they had said 'I am the expert, I know'. This provokes feelings among the group members. Some will react as children to a parent, some as pupils to a teacher, some as a team to its captain. Some of the feelings will be warm and positive but some will be negative because no one really likes to be organized. Both the group leader and the members draw upon their previous experiences of groups which will include their own families for role models in their ways of working together. They tend to remember the limitations of those early groups and to attribute characteristics of their members to those of the present group. Thus a member may see the leader as a bossy parent, a bully, or a disagreeable schoolteacher. While the good and benevolent characteristics of past colleagues have their own influence, unfortunately it is the less commendable behaviour that is remembered and often initiated so the leader who is unsure of herself may reproduce the authoritarian behaviour of a teacher even though she had resented the same treatment meted out to her at school. This phenomenon of new groups will pass if the group has an immediate task, while the members are working together each will reveal his strengths and weaknesses, gaining an identity within the group that will generate its own responses replacing the fantasy reactions of the early meetings.

The recognition of each other as people with different contributions is an important aspect of group interaction. People fear not being valued by others, or given credit for what they do. They need respect and courtesy. If members do not think they are being treated properly in a group they will first stop talking and then stop coming. It is also necessary for them to believe that the group's purposes are worthwhile and likely to be fulfilled. Each member gives up some freedom to attend meetings. To have to do something regularly turns it from a pleasure into work. Those who carry responsibilities within the group, such as secretary or teamaker, have a greater obligation to attend regularly and they need a deeper commitment than other members as well as a constant expression of the group's approval for whatever they do in order to sustain them week by week.

The nurse who initiates a self-help group is not a member of the group in the true sense as she has no shared condition or problem. In her capacity as resource person she should act as hostess to the group, encouraging participation, but leaving it to the members to share experiences, define their problems and seek solutions together. If the group needs expert help they can be helped to find it but if they are to develop as a self-help group they must be responsible jointly for the group activities.

SOME CRITERIA FOR ASSESSING GOOD GROUP WORK

1. The atmosphere should be informal, comfortable and relaxed so that there is neither tension nor boredom.

2. Most members should contribute to the discussions.

3. The purpose of the group should be agreed by all members.

4. Members should listen to one another. They may not always agree but disagreement is friendly, there is no tyrant trying to impose ideas on the majority. When there is disagreement there is not hasty decision taking and the many do not override the interests of the few.

5. Most agreement should be reached by concensus.

6. Criticism should be frank but not personal.

7. Feelings as well as ideas should be freely expressed.

8. The group should not be dominated by the leader, leadership may pass from one member to another; there should be little evidence of a struggle for power.

9. When action needs to be taken a clear allocation of tasks should be made and accepted.

10. The group is self-critical.

THE FAMILY AS A GROUP

The family group is one in which most group processes can be observed. The members show a group identity, they have special roles and complex interactions. Every family develops its own communication networks, has its own values and has its own group culture. The family identity originates from the following:

1. They initiate or have some memory of a common household.

2. Every family has a shared history which includes births, deaths, separations, illnesses and crises associated with both pain and joy.

3. In most cases there is a cohesiveness between family members although they have separate identities. Each individual may be quite different in attitudes and behaviour when apart from the family group.

4. The family has a group attitude to the outside world, feeling it to be friendly, hostile, wicked, hypocritical or foolish.

5. Families have ideals, ambitions and goals held in common.

INTERACTION IN FAMILIES

Within each family system there are subgroups, each with their own ways of reacting to each other and to the whole group. Parents, for example, are a subgroup with particular authority over certain expenditure, over discipline and generally over behaviour within the home. Mother and daughters may constitute a subgroup. So may all the children together when young and at certain times in later years, as for example when they reunite to plan a celebration for their parents' golden wedding or to help when they are ill. The family as a whole will not find it necessary for members to make their feelings known explicitly but will share complex non-verbal communication patterns; their speech will often reveal an interfamily vocabulary, a humour and a teasing style that is very exclusive. It may not include the sons- and daughters-in-law. Thus when the married members of a family return to their parents' home in times of crisis, the communication may involve many crossed currents between the brothers' and sisters' old style of interaction and the family communication patterns which they severally have developed with their spouses and their own children.

Each member of the family has many roles, the husband is also father, he may be breadwinner, gardener, car owner and disciplinarian. The roles and the behaviour expected of people in those roles is recognized throughout the family. Fathers do not cry, mother's job is to have meals ready, brothers don't tell tales.

Authority patterns will vary between families. They may be patriarchal, matriarchal or democratic, according to the leadership and control exerted. The handling of conflict in a family is unique. Ideas develop about what is right and wrong as well as what sanctions should be imposed upon those who break the rules. The family as a whole will have feelings about work, poverty, health, as well as society and its institutions which will affect the way in which they receive and work with doctors, nurses, home helps and other caring individuals.

Not all family relationships are happy and harmonious, some jealousies and dislikes are profoundly destructive. Sometimes, however, relatives who have quarrelled bitterly are as devastated by terminal illness and bereavement as if they had loved one another dearly.

THE ASSESSMENT OF THE FAMILY SITUATION

This should be undertaken on two levels, by examining the family as a collection of separate individuals and as a group. Each person will have strengths and weaknesses, defences and vulnerabilities. Within the family they will have roles, relationships and ways of coping with a crisis that may help or hinder them when they have to contend with illness. A son who is cosseted by his own wife and who does little in his own home may come back when his mother is sick to clean and shop for her. Financial hardship, poverty or chronic illness may be seen as a failure by some families when the breadwinner has to give up work, but the individual members may not be lacking in sensitivity to the patient in his troubles.

There is one form of family pathology that should be recognized if it occurs, that is scapegoating. In order to achieve or maintain the unity of a group it may be necessary to have a deviant member who is held responsible for the group tensions. This may be an elderly patient but it may not, sometimes it is a child within the family. The child of a patient with multiple sclerosis may be accused of staying out late, mixing in bad company, avoiding his mother, refusing to help in the home. In the end he may do these things. The parents worry about the child, not realizing that their anxieties drive him to do the very thing they worry about, because worrying over the child is less frightening to them than having to face the problems of the physical deterioration in the patient.

Bromley[9] describes the averse properties of old age, because the appearance and behaviour of the elderly is different from what is generally regarded as normal, people with little direct contact with older people are sometimes filled with a sense of horror and distaste when they see them. Thus when an elderly person comes into a household some negative feelings may be released, his presence felt to be a constraint and he is thought to be the cause of problems between other members of the family.

If this happens it is difficult to integrate the elderly person into the family and to be isolated or denied implicit approval in a family group can be more difficult to tolerate than when one is alone and lonely. It is sometimes preferable for an elderly woman to live alone in squalor than to live in luxury with a daughter-in-law who cannot bear her to go into the kitchen even to make a cup of tea in case she makes it dirty or breaks a cup.

THE STAFF GROUP OR WORK GROUP

This group differs from the self-help group because membership is compulsory. There may be both formal and informal contact between members, but decision making usually takes place in subgroups and when ratified by the seniors is conveyed to the others in formal meetings for final agreement. The formal meetings may have a chairman and an agenda. To some degree a staff group resembles a large family, nicknames are often given to the senior members that imply a parental relationship but they also denote the role and responsibility the leader is expected to assume. Information circulates within the group and when this is confidential to members it is often referred to as being 'kept in the family'. The less senior members may behave in the same way as siblings do, indulging in friendly rivalry and vying for the favours of those in authority. Such comparisons can be carried too far, however, the staff group has a task to perform and each member of the work group has a particular role and responsibilities. They also have a professional as well as a personal identity which will modify their behaviour.

Klein[7] identifies several roles that may be adopted by group members, some often met in staff groups are:

1. The expert who is the information giver on whom others come to depend for clarification of facts.
2. The facilitator who is able to help others contribute to the group and make them feel that their offering is worthwhile.
3. The co-ordinator is the constructive member who can bring order to

the discussions, reconciling different viewpoints and resolving conflicts when they arise.

4. The morale booster is able to support others in the group and maintain their enthusiasm.

5. Opinion leaders may be the most able, know the right people, be popular or have in the past made several sensible recommendations. They are the influential members who, when they give ideas or state opinions, will be supported by others.

6. There are the agreers, those who will support the opinion leader and seek to work with them.

7. There may be an isolate, who if she is fortunate will be neglected but tolerated in the group. Denied communication she may still find satisfaction in pretending to be part of the group, alternatively she may be rejected by the members even though she tries to reach out to them.

Generally a person needs the group acceptance and they try to gain it by behaving in a manner acceptable to the other members. Members are seen as friendly when they express ideas the rest approve of and unfriendly when their attitudes are withdrawn or hostile, or when they refuse to share their ideas with others.

Individuals in the staff group are often faced with conflict situations, often comprising of:

1. *Authority problems*

When one of the team needs to be defiant and show off.

2. *Dependency problems*

When a member behaves like a child, depending upon the seniors for guidance, not wanting to share with others the responsibility for either group decision making or maintaining the group processes. This can cause chaos in a busy practice team when it is a relatively senior person who abdicates their responsibilities, allows another member to make decisions alone, that should be made by common agreement.

3. *Resistance to sharing*

Change sometimes threatens the particular individual's autonomy or constrains her activities. When a member of the staff group has found a comfortable way of working they may resent any sort of inovations, they may not want to see any new members join the group in case their ideas are disruptive. They may even oppose the suggestion that the time of the group meetings be changed. These are generally people who want approval from the group but who do not want to become involved in the joint work. They frequently look back to a golden age rather than forward to a new era, and are exceedingly difficult to work with.

4. *The idiosyncratic colleague*

This is the person who has always to have their needs met regardless of the needs of others and can, therefore, impede the group's activities. Present at meetings only because they must attend, they cannot see anyone else's point of view. Outside the group they may discuss their ideas as if they were acceptable to all the group members which is irritating for the others and frequently causes misunderstandings.

It is sometimes possible for the group to talk through the particular behaviour that is disrupting their work. There are four aspects to behaviour:[8]

	Known to self	Not known to self
Known to others	[1] [Known to all]	[2] [Unconscious but observed by others]
Not known to others	[3] [Hidden]	[4] [Unconscious and unrecognized]

Fig. 6. The four aspects of behaviour.

1. The aspect that we recognize in our selves and other people are aware of it.

2. Behaviour that others observe in us, which is not apparent to us.

3. Information that we have about our behaviour but which we do not choose to share with others.

4. That part of ourselves of which neither we nor anyone else has any conscious knowledge.

The aim of any discussion must be to extend 1. into 2. and 3. If we can, with sensitivity, tell others how we see them behaving in certain circumstances they may then do the same for us. They may notice that we become agitated if there is dissention in the group, or become defensive when certain criticisms are voiced. With increasing self-knowledge we may act with more concern and understanding. If the group members feel secure enough in their relationships one with another they may be able to talk at a group meeting about their feelings for each other and the behaviour that troubles them, the person may be able to modify their ways of working, and in consequence the whole team act more constructively together.

UNDERSTANDING VULNERABILITY

To be vulnerable is to be susceptible to injury, not proof against hurt, criticism, etc. This definition is extended by health and social workers to include those susceptible to disease and injury, resulting from infection, trauma, degeneration, as well as such social factors as loneliness and cold. All are vulnerable at times, when criticized, afraid or alone. Vulnerability increases with dependency. The child, the handicapped person, and the elderly are more often at risk and face more hazards than others do. Some environments increase the risk of emotional, physical or social disease. Fatigue, hunger and cold reduce resistance to disease and increase the likelihood of initiating behaviour that would antagonize others, or limit a person's capacity to tolerate ideas that are at variance with his own.

In different societies and at different times, certain people will be seen as vulnerable and therefore in need of protection. It is not easy to know how to use the concept of vulnerability in predicting 'at risk' groups in a caseload. When in 1965 an 'at risk' register was started for infants having certain antenatal or birth experiences in common, it was thought possible to predict which children might develop handicapping conditions. In the event, so many could be considered vulnerable that the register had no predictive value. Yet there are patients and care-givers in any caselist that are more susceptible to injury or illness than average and every district nurse has to make special arrangements to supervise them more closely. Although most domiciliary patients, because they are elderly, dependent upon others, and handicapped in some way, are easily hurt by careless words or deeds. Some groups such as the recently bereaved, the depressed, patients with sensory deprivation and patients living with insensitive relatives are always at risk, as are the relatives of the mentally ill and those who have a dying patient to care for.[9]

What general principles then should indicate the need for close surveillance? Domiciliary patients' vulnerability arises from one or more factors, either it is circumstantial, i.e. because of the death of a relative or perhaps the change of home help. It may be caused by physical deterioration: sensory deprivation, increasing deafness or loss of sight for instance. It may also be the result of inadequate interaction, when relatives or neighbours do not visit, or when they do not listen or talk about things that are important to the patient.

The first priority should be to ensure, wherever possible, that every patient has some contact with an adult who is able to recognize when help is needed and get it. The nurse has the responsibility to assess in each case whether such a person is available, or could be found and would be acceptable to the patient, to form a network between the patient and the health and social services. The quality of the relationship between the patient and the contact is important. Some may be reliable in assessing physical health but are not sensitive to emotional need. Some may alternate between kindness and criticism and are not, therefore, always as supportive as they might be. It may be that given time the nurse can help them in their role. Alternatively she may have to supplement their observation by visiting herself more frequently than the clinical condition warrants.

The worker who can recognize his own vulnerability has a useful yardstick to measure the pain it causes, but like any painful condition vulnerability may be denied. Some people regard it as weakness and if so there is the risk that they will deny that which they believe to be an imperfection within themselves. Because this denial is an unconscious process it is not easily recognized by the worker herself or colleagues working with her. It can, nevertheless, act as a block when it comes to helping people cope with their own problems. 'I am deaf and I don't feel that everyone is talking about me' is no way to start persuading a deaf patient to overcome her paranoia.

The patient who is terminally ill may want to know what is happening to him yet dread to hear the fatal diagnosis. The nurse may respond to his desire for knowledge thinking she herself would want to know the truth, but would she in all circumstances? Certainly some people would want to know more than they would want not to be told, but all are ambivalent to some extent. It is a sensitive nurse who can appreciate the relative fluctuations of mood, report them accurately, and with the doctor and close relatives who are responsible for the patient's comfort, she can plan what to say about prognosis during the last weeks of life.

REFERENCES

1. ATKINSON, H. (1967). *Introduction to psychology*, 4th ed., New York: Harcourt Brace & World.
2. ATKINSON, H. (1967). *Introduction to psychology*, 4th ed., New York: Harcourt Brace & World.
3. ERIKSON, E.H. (1963). Childhood Society. Harmondsworth: Penguin.
4. THOMAS CHESS and BIRCH The origins of personality.
5. MASLOW, A.H. (1954). *Motivation and personality*. New York: Harper & Row.
   MASLOW, A.H. (1962). *Towards a psychology of being*. New York: Harper & Row.
6. ROGERS, G.R. *A theory of personality and behaviour*. Reprinted in Social Behaviour and Experience. Burns & Stevens. 1975.
7. KLEIN, T. (1967). *Working with Groups*. London: Hutchinson.
8. WALKER, M., & SMITH, G. The art of knowing oneself within the team. *Health and Social Service Journal*. December 7th, 1979.
9. BROMLEY, D.B. Speculations in Social Environmental Gerontology. *Nursing Times*, April 21st 1977.

FURTHER READING

ATKINSON, H. (1967). Introduction to psychology. New York: Harcourt Brace & World.
Open University Social Psychology D305. Block 7. *Integration and the Concept of Self*.
Open University Social Psychology D308. Block 8. *Social Perception*.
JAMES, D.E. (1975). *Introduction to psychology*. London: Panther.
RADDOCK, R. (1969). *Roles and Relationships*. London: Routledge & Kegan Paul.

CHAPTER 6

Communication and Counselling Interviews

Communication is a process by which people come to understand others and are in turn understood by them. Good communication is the basis of good nursing practice and proper team work. It facilitates understanding of the policies and regulations issued within any health authority, and ensures that the reports and records of individual members of staff are compiled into an accurate picture of home nursing care.

Communication begins at birth. The young dependent child is restless and feeds less well when his mother is agitated. This in turn causes her increased anxiety which probably upsets the child even more, and sets up a vicious circle of stress. Babies are usually more robust than inexperienced mothers think and they settle quickly once a contented rhythm is established. Nevertheless the mother needs all her vitality, ingenuity and patience to meet such minor crises and it is always better if they can be prevented. This early experience of communication within a close personal relationship demonstrates how attuned people have to become to others in order to ensure good communication. In time the child learns to assess his mother's moods from her expression, the way in which she holds him and the tone of her voice as she comforts or chides him. These clues are known as non-verbal communication, they are frequently made unintentionally and are the first and most basic form of interaction. Communication without words appears less important once speech and language are developed but it remains the way in which thoughts, emotions and feelings are transmitted, and in conversation gestures are a very useful adjunct to the spoken word.[1]

Some messages are direct and specific, others are unconscious. Serious misunderstanding may occur when a spoken message is contradicted by unintended signals. When a nurse reassures a patient his anxiety is not likely to be allayed if her face and posture denote tension as she works and he is aware of her unspoken concern.

Patients frequently are left to build up a picture of their illness and their prognosis from what is left unsaid, and from the non-verbal clues the staff give. Nurses and doctors are not always good communicators. They do not volunteer much information and often they evade any but the most superficial discussion of the patient's problems, particularly when the prognosis is uncertain and complete recovery is unlikely.

Some communication is essential for mental health. In old age, when hearing fails, facial expressions, signs and touch may be the most significant and meaningful method of interaction left to patients. Friends and relatives need to be told this and helped to express concern and affection in this manner until the end of the patient's life.

PROCESS RECORDING

Successful communication as an integral part of nursing care does not just happen but is a learned skill. Analysing various interactions will enable the student to recognize when barriers are inhibiting the conversation or words and signals are misunderstood. The process recording may be used as a tool to assess the nurse/patient interaction. It is a verbatim recording, to the extent that memory permits, of the verbal and non-verbal messages that have passed between the nurse, the patient and the family. It should include:

1. A written record of the verbal and behavioural communication in the sequence in which it occurred between the participants.
2. Written comments identifying the feeling the nurse experiences and those she believes were experienced by the patient.
3. The nurse's written analysis and evaluation of the meaning of the interaction and the clues to the patient's needs.

Through observing the words used by each person the learner may achieve a growing awareness and ultimately an understanding of her own expressions. She will learn to what extent she controls the conversation and how much she permits the patient to express his personal concerns.

The act of writing down an interaction in such detail is time consuming and sometimes tedious, particularly if done thoroughly. Each process recording should be studied systematically and purposefully, the learner concentrating on such aspects as:

1. The broad range of verbal communication during a visit.

2. Her questions.
3. The words used by the patient.
4. The appropriateness of her responses to the patient's words.
5. The silences.
6. The non-verbal clues.

The nurse's conversation may for example be studied in terms of the questions she asks: are they phrased in such a way either to invite or to inhibit the patient's response. Questions prefaced by 'why' may tend to put the patient on the defensive because they ask him to reveal the motivation for his feelings and behaviour. Some questions elicit an elaborate response but sentences beginning with a form of the verb *to be* tend to result in a monosyllabic answer.

With practice the record keeper will be aware not only of the words spoken but the intonation and modulation of the voice, and she will notice to what extent these are consistent with the words used. The words of a relative may suggest happiness for example but the tone may convey sadness and great concern.

While the spoken comments tend to be to some degree in accord with the expectations of the listener, much of what is thought and felt is revealed through varying movements in the position of the body or parts of the body. The nurse will know what she is feeling and be able to relate this directly to her posture or movements. She can, however, only impute feelings to another. She may observe the overt manifestation of the activity of the autonomic nervous system, the patient's colour may change from slight to deep pallor, from slight to extensive flushing, his hands may be damp or tightly clasped. The nurse can suggest these feelings to him in an open ended question such as 'You feel angry about . . .', 'You are worried in case . . .', or 'You are sorry you said . . .'. The patient may then confirm that the feelings were the ones he was experiencing at that moment and may be able to share with the nurse the causes of his distress.

It is useful and interesting to study non-verbal responses with a patient who for physical or emotional reasons is unable to use verbal communication, or to analyse the communication problems that may be experienced by the family of a patient with Parkinson's disease whose expressionless face and shaking hands inhibit his non-verbal signs.

As the nurse studies the written record of the process of communication there is an opportunity to reassess her own behaviour, attitudes and feelings. She may become aware that she avoids responding to some of the patient's statements, or that at times she overwhelms him with inappropriate information. Sometimes she may find that she changes the subject whenever certain topics are mentioned.

In analysing the interaction in sequence the learner should question what events initiated which spoken comments, what words, phrases or gestures guided the process. The student's theoretical background in social and behavioural studies will contribute to the depth and breadth of her knowledge about her own and her patient's behaviour and attitudes, but she will need help from her practical teacher if she is going to develop fully her understanding of interpersonal relationship skills. The teacher's function is to guide the student through the analysis of the process and encourage her to try new approaches.

The student may recognize the patient's fear but not feel comfortable enough herself to broach the subject. She may find it helpful to discuss with her teacher how she could open up the conversation and help the patient share the problems he is feeling. She may need support in order to accept the emotions that are directed against her which may be very threatening. She may need help to overcome the tendency to ward off expressions of anger or dissatisfaction when things get difficult by offering praise or flattery. Too much sweetness, too much sympathy, too quick a reassurance can disarm a patient and prevent him from coming to terms with the underlying cause of his distress.

Success in such an interaction is a gratifying experience not only for the nurse but also for the patient who feels that at last his problems are being understood by those who care for him. Then together nurse and patient may begin to explore ways in which the difficulties can be overcome.

THE PROCESS OF COMMUNICATION

When a simple message is passed between two people the process can be broken down into six stages:

1. The intention to transmit the message.
2. Finding the words to express the idea accurately and lucidly.
3. Deciding how the message should be sent, whether in the form of a written report, by telephone, or during an informal chat over a cup of coffee.
4. The second person will receive or block the message.
5. If he receives the message he will interpret it in the light of his previous experience and knowledge.
6. He will accept or reject it wholly or in part, and respond accordingly.

The process is complicated and inhibited by the thoughts, emotions, prejudices and needs of all concerned. They occasionally block all communication between people as in some psychiatric disorders but more frequently they interfere with and distort the messages as they are passed.

BARRIERS TO COMMUNICATION

Barriers to communication include:

1. The perceived status of the speaker.
2. The language used.
3. Internal factors such as anxiety or anger.
4. Extrinsic factors such as distraction and noise.
5. Expectations, generally resulting from previous experience.
6. Misinterpretation of gestures, sometimes the result of cultural differences.

The problems of authority frequently distort communication. Some people, once they have attributed authority to another, will unquestioningly follow their teaching, others will resist anything they regard as imposing a way of working upon them. A patient with a strange skin condition was questioned about his diet by his doctor. The question was framed thus: 'Is your diet normal?', and the answer was 'Yes'. When the nurse visited she too asked what he has eaten during the day and he told her he had two ounces of milk every two hours. She then discovered that twenty years before, when he went to the local hospital complaining of epigastric pain, a nurse had told him to take two ounces of milk two hourly, and this he had done. His skin condition and general weakness were finally diagnosed as scurvy. He had attributed authority to the nurse at the hospital and followed her instructions without question. He had misunderstood the meaning of the word 'normal' when it was used by his doctor in relation to his diet. The doctor had intended to ask whether his diet contained the range of nutrients needed to maintain health. The patient interpreted it as meaning normal for him, that is not significantly changed within the past few weeks.

Words which are emotionally charged can obscure the meaning of a sentence, particularly if the hearer comes to a conclusion based not only on the factual meaning but upon the emotions aroused by the words. While the use of emotional words in writing is condemned it is common in speech. Sometimes it is a symptom of a deeper malaise, 'emotional thinking'. The term 'dirty old man' has from time to time been attributed to a patient whose only fault was to yearn to touch the friendly, attractive young woman who was perhaps the only visitor to the house who had any time for him. Reporting factual information only in descriptions of patients and their environments helps to avoid emotional thinking. Value judgements rarely add to the store of information on which an assessment should be based. They may prejudice another care-giver against the patient preventing the development of a helping relationship between them, and such remarks may be libellous.

UNACCEPTABLE MESSAGES

Only certain aspects of messages are acceptable, that which is not is dealt with in one of several ways. They may be disregarded. If no response at all is given when a message is received it is as though there had been no message. The patient who hates being dependent upon his sister may ignore those remarks that seem to him to imply that they are managing well. The nurse who unwittingly says 'How fortunate you are to have your sister to look after you' may be surprised to find her remark received in stony silence. The patient who objects to the home help's familiarity may ignore her cheery greeting. Sometimes the rejection is more profound and the unacceptable part of the message may not even be recognized. Thus a patient with cancer may deny that he was ever told about either his diagnosis or his prognosis although he asked for this information. The patient told to lose weight may believe that the doctor wanted him to eat well to keep up his strength.

It is often difficult to tell whether unacceptable messages are not recognized for what they are, or whether they are disregarded and forgotten immediately. The patient whose visit is postponed due to other more urgent work may at the time agree to wait, but when the nurse arrives later he may be angry and protest that he knew nothing of the changed arrangement. Fault may lie within the person sending the message, the message itself may lack clarity, all misunderstandings are not due to emotional blocks in the recipient. Responsibility for analysing the interaction, anticipating and wherever possible preventing errors in communication, must rest with the professional person involved.[2]

The nurse therefore is the key person in communications involving the patient and his family and is as responsible as any other professional person in the interdisciplinary communication within the primary health care team.

ORGANIZATIONAL COMMUNICATION

While interpersonal relationships are based on direct exchanges and take place when people meet together, write to one another or speak by telephone, organizational communication is frequently more formal and indirect. When policy documents are circulated through the authority, the response should be made equally formally to the policy maker. If no response is made the wrong policy may be implemented by default. It is useless to grumble with one's peers about a regulation from the DHSS. The right way to respond is through a professional association. Comments from small groups carry less weight than those made through professional organizations and trade unions. In official communications knowing the right channel is as important as selecting the right words if it is hoped to influence policies or change the direction in which events are moving.

In organizations information is power. It follows therefore that communication is a powerful tool that puts information into certain people's hands, and by withholding it from others can deprive them of influence. A study of any working group will reveal various patterns of communication both formal and informal. Within a primary health care team there will be networks through which information passes. There may be a diary in which all staff put their fixed appointments each week, yet the receptionist may be the only person who always knows what is happening and where everyone is at any time. The doctor may share his medical journal with the health visitor who may not always remember to pass it on to the district nurse.

Within every organization some form of written communication exists as a record of work done. This is true of the district nursing service. Some of the most important are the reports submitted and the records kept by the fieldworkers. Official records are written facts and reports are extensions of records in which facts are interpreted and decisions communicated to others who are also caring for the patients. Reports may be given verbally, or telephoned into the centres in the first place, but should also be written. Oral evidence supported by detailed legible and presentable notes is likely to be accepted in a court of law and may win the day. Inadequate or absent notes may force an out-of-court settlement of a claim which otherwise might have been defended.

The validity of records is undermined if they are inaccurate, written in insufficient detail, or if they contain irrelevant material. Most important they should be written at the time of the treatment, with no erasures or mutilations, dated, and signed with a full signature. Records should document the following facts about patient care:

1. The original message, how it was received, what day and at what time it was received.
2. The patient's details: name, address and age.
3. The diagnosis, treatment and other orders.
4. Day-to-day progress of the acutely ill, or weekly review of the long-term sick.
5. A record of all drugs given, dated — with time of administration and a full signature.

The most important function of records is to enable the team to provide the patient with consistent care. The written case notes are the only continuous record of what was or was not done. A well documented episode of illness may be used in teaching students as the success or failure of the methods of treament should be recorded. Researchers make extensive use of patients' records.

The forms submitted to the authority giving a summary of work undertaken enables nurse managers to estimate and if necessary adjust the work undertaken by various nursing teams, to make a case for new staff, and to submit an accurate account annually of the public money that is spent on the service. Epidemiologists too gather statistics from medical and nursing records, identifying the health status of special communities and of different age groups.

Reports are written to be read. Busy people read with varying degrees of concentration. Records should therefore be legible, written in short sentences and be as concise as is consistent with accuracy. They should be set out in a straightforward manner and presented as logically as possible.

Reports are frequently read by patients and their relatives when they are left in the patient's home. Such reports must be written with this in mind, being full enough to demonstrate that you do know what is happening to the patient without causing him offence or agitation.

Reports that are read by strangers, for example those sent to a consultant in an outpatient department, must contain sufficient information to enable him to appreciate the significance of the observations made or the recommendations suggested.

Any reader will have his own set of expectations and ambiguous sentences will be seen by the reader as confirmation of his own ideas. It is important to make certain that the presentation is as clear and straightforward as possible.

Patient records do not belong to the patient, the nurse or the local authority. Legally their ownership rests with the Secretary of State. The patient however does have the right to know who has access to the notes, and whoever has custody of those notes must ensure that neither the record nor its contents are communicated to anyone not authorized to receive the information. There are occasions when disclosure is required by law. A nurse can be compelled on a subpoena or a witness summons to disclose what she knows about a patient. A solicitor acting on behalf of a patient may demand medical or nursing information. All notes passed from one doctor to another or one nurse to another is generally done with the patient's implied consent. However the patient would be within his rights to ask to see the notes that were being passed and to be told what they meant. When records are accessible to many members of the caring team and are a communication tool in the practice there may be a contradiction between communication and confidentiality. Confidentiality is an issue that must be kept under careful review at all times.

THE COUNSELLING INTERVIEW

District nurses are not counsellors, but as they work with individuals and families in distress they have to be able to help people to express their thoughts, feelings and emotions, and offer to them a supportive relationship through which they can work towards solving their problems, albeit only partially, or come to terms with those situations that cannot be changed. The skills in this helping process are based on the same principles that underly all counselling and are a modification of the responses and reactions common to all social interaction. It is a particularly sensitive form of communication in which the person needing help is always vulnerable and the person offering help has to meet emotional demands that come not only from the patient or family needing counsel but from the process itself. It demands an intellectual and emotional honesty, an understanding of oneself as well as an understanding of other people.

THE PRINCIPLES OF COUNSELLING

The principles underlying the counselling interview can be stated very simply, but their application is complex and difficult. They stem from a belief in the worth of each individual. Belief in this fundamental tenet makes it possible to accept people as they are, with all their strengths and weaknesses, without criticism either of their way of life, or condemnation of their beliefs and values. It will also underly the principle that people are entitled to make their own decisions and be responsible for their own affairs. The patient, the relative, another colleague, or anyone who turns to the nurse for help has a right to expect that his privacy will be respected and that his affairs will never be revealed inappropriately to another. Where there is no trust and no confidence very little help will be received. Although the intentions of the helper may be good, the relationship through which she must work is fundamentally flawed.

The helping relationship also depends upon the person in need seeing benefit that may be derived from the process and feeling that the help is appropriate to his problems. An agreement to work together is important, help cannot be given without the consent, freely given, by the person in need. Of course much helping is simple. Most patients know that they need certain treatment in order to recover, or that because of heart failure they must change their life style in order to enjoy several more years of living, and they accept the discomfort and the problems that are involved with as good a grace as they can and make the best of it.

Sometimes a patient cannot accept the limitations of his disease. The young diabetic boy for example finds balancing insulin, diet and exercise unacceptable, and wants to enjoy the present with his friends, eating and drinking what he fancies, turning night into day, dancing until the early hours, letting the future take care of itself. Such a young man needs professional counselling, but in order that he presents to the social worker having a mind to be helped the nurse will have to use all her skills of helpful persuasion. She will have to support the parents who will no doubt in their distress alternate between begging him to be sensible and threatening him with dire consequences if he doesn't. In these situations the nurse needs the same skills as the counsellor, as well as her knowledge of the pathological condition and the physiological changes that accompany it. She must understand the problems of accepting long term illness. She must not underestimate the difficulties facing the boy as he passes through adolescence and needs to be one with his peers: nor those of the parents who watch him risking his well-being and his life.

THE HELPING RELATIONSHIP

In what circumstances is a helping relationship created? Over the years it has been shown that a relationship in which there is trust, confidence and consistency is one that is most helpful. How then can the nurse behave in such a way as to be seen as trustworthy, dependent and consistent? There are certain external arrangements that are important such as keeping appointments, allowing sufficient time, concentrating on the matter in hand and respecting confidences. The person who has to wait for a counselling interview will find him or herself getting irritable, anxious and impatient, all emotions that tend to inhibit the desire to share with the counsellor. It is necessary therefore to visit by arrangement when counselling is likely to be a primary activity during the visit, or to be at the Centre at a prearranged time, when a room can be made available and the conversation can be carried on without interruption for as long as necessary.

The helper has to examine how she feels about the person needing help and the circumstances in which he finds himself. If she is annoyed with the other person, mistrustful or critical, it is very difficult to hide these feelings and yet they are likely to be sensed by the other and interpreted as inconsistencies. It is not easy to maintain a relationship knowing that one's own feelings are likely to disrupt it at any time. The helper had better be honest with herself and the other person involved, accepting whatever feelings are being experienced without denying their importance or playing down the problems they present. This open attitude is usually recognized as genuine and interpreted as dependable. When the helper is unaware of the feelings that she is experiencing, as is sometimes the case, then the communication contains contradictory messages. This confuses the listener and makes him distrustful even though he may be unaware of the actual source of the difficulty. If therefore through defensiveness one is not prepared to heed what is within oneself, successful helping through a counselling interview is not likely to take place.

Few people listen to what others are saying. Generally they are frantically trying to think what to say when the other falls silent. The more sensitive the subject matter the more difficult it is to listen and this is very true when nurse and relative together try to anticipate the problems that will follow the death of a patient. It is the nurse who must adjust her contribution to meet the needs of the relatives, if she fails to speak to them in terms they can respond to she has not developed a helping relationship at all. She must be able to experience and show positive attitudes towards the person, attitudes of warmth, caring, liking, interest and respect. It is not easy. We are often afraid that if we show these attitudes we may become trapped by them, people might make depends upon us, or we may be disappointed in our trust, so we tend to seek a 'professional' attitude or an impersonal relationship. This bears no relationship to whether we call the relative by her first name or an affectionate substitute such as 'dear'. It depends upon our relationship with ourselves. Accepting our own feelings and insecurities increases the likelihood that we can establish a helping relationship with another. Knowing ourselves and permitting this to show through to another is a most difficult task, but it is necessary if we are to see others for what they are, accept them and relate to them. Once this first hurdle is recognized there is another in order to make the relationship truly a helpful one. The person helping must learn how to understand the feelings of the other to be able to project her personality into the situation and to comprehend it fully. It is not sympathy. Sympathy is experiencing the same emotion. It is empathy which is getting into another's world, his feelings and personal thoughts, seeing it as he does, experiencing it so completely that there is no desire to evaluate or judge it. Even a minimal amount of this understanding is helpful, a bumbling and faulty attempt to catch the confused complexity of the person's meaning is helpful. There is no doubt though that it is most helpful when the counsellor can see and formulate clearly the meaning of the other's experiences that until then had for him been unclear and bewildering.

Arising from this is another consideration. The helper must have an independence from the other person and his predicament. She must be strong enough not to be cast down by his depression, frightened by his fear, destroyed by his anger or enslaved by his dependency. Only if she is separate enough can she accept him without wanting to change him wholly or partially to a model of her making.

THE ORGANIZATION OF A COUNSELLING INTERVIEW

The counselling interview is a conversation within a particular context that has a specific purpose, the pattern of which is directed by the nurse. She may have as her purpose, to obtain information, to give information, to create a more positive attitude to a problem or to support a person through a long term problem. The other person should share her purpose though may not express it in great detail until they understand each other thoroughly.

The scene will be set for the interview so that as far as possible both are comfortable, relaxed and unlikely to be uninterrupted. Counselling is not exclusively a nurse/patient activity, the use of the word patient in this context means the person receiving counsel.

The first objective of the nurse must be to establish rapport between them, making certain that the other knows what he is there for, the nature of the help that is offered and its limits.

Once the interview has begun, using such general remarks as 'How do you feel about . . .' she will endeavour to explore the problems that are caused by the situation that has arisen. Meanwhile she will watch for behavioural evidence that will either confirm or refute what is being said. Avoiding any signs of approval or disapproval she will reflect whatever is said to her back to the patient in order that he may verify his own attitudes and see more clearly what he can do to help himself and others, or understand what underlies his inability to cope with his circumstances.

Feelings may be reflected in the following way. The feelings that appear to the nurse to be implicit in any statement made to her can be reflected back to the patient in the nurse's own words. This does not mean mimicking or repeating like an echo, but saying, 'You feel angry about . . .', 'You must worry when . . .', 'You must feel sorry you can't . . .'. The important result is the association between the statement made and how the patient felt about it. A feeling that he may or may not have recognized before. An elderly patient cared for by a rather trying sister said one day 'Oh, I wish she were dead'. 'Do you really hate her as much as that?' said the nurse. 'No, I don't suppose I do' said the patient slowly, looking rather shamefaced, but she added after a moment's pause, 'How do I know what I mean until I hear myself saying it?'

The interviewer may find it helpful to preface her remarks with such general statement as 'You feel . . .', 'You think . . .'. She must of course be sure that both she and the patient are using a common vocabulary and understand each other's meaning. It is better to formulate as statements any remarks and phrases that might cause confusion.

The nurse must be able to wait through the pauses until there is a response. Once a response has been made it should be accepted. Only the emotion most recently expressed should be reflected, going back to a situation missed or mishandled is not helpful. When inconsistencies are expressed they should be noted but not challenged. Decisions, solutions and constructive ideas should be reflected back to the patient only when they have predominated in the conversation for some minutes over such emotions as hostility, fear, insecurity or such feelings as confusion and bewilderment.

While allowing the patient plenty of time to reply, watch for significant remarks. This requires complete attention. It may be that what is left unsaid is as important as what is said. Notice which topics cause embarrassment. While the patient is speaking he may be encouraged by neutral sounds such as 'Mm' or 'Ahhah'. However it is most important that false meaning should not be attributed to these sounds and in circumstances where smiles and nods are taken as to express approval some other more appropriate neutral gesture must be substituted.

Time is not elastic. Were it so district nurses would be justified in spending many hours counselling in the course of their duties. They must, however, be selective in what they do and refer those patients who need intensive care to others who can devote more time to the task, and who have had intensive training to develop the special skills needed to work at greater depth. The district nurse with a busy caseload must calculate how long she can spend with any particular patient without jeopardizing others who also need her attention. It may be that a counselling interview can only last 10–15 minutes, in which case the patient should know at the start and should be warned when the time is nearly finished. Ending an interview is never easy. Occasionally it has to be prolonged because of the nature of the problem but the promise of a further discussion or of referral to someone with different pressures of work will generally help the person to trust the nurse and use the help of a colleague. In each interview there is usually only time to re-establish the relationship and explore one idea superficially.

Once the nurse has mastered the basic skills she will be able to use the whole visit for patient counselling. As she carries out her nursing duties she will be able to help the patient and sometimes such other care-givers as may be in the room working with her to look frankly at their problems and the feelings they have about them.

REFERENCES

1. BYRTON, L. (1975). *The Family Life of Sick Children*. London: Routledge & Kegan Paul.
2. HARRISON, S.P. (1977). *Families in Stress*. London: Royal College of Nursing.

FURTHER READING

COMMUNICATION

HARGREAVES, David H. (1975). *Interpersonal Relations and Education*. London: Routledge & Kegan Paul.
JOHNSON, Abercrombie K.L. (1960). *The Anatomy of Judgement*. Harmondsworth: Penguin.
RUDDOCK, Ralph. (1969). *Roles and Relationships*. London: Routledge & Kegan Paul.

RECORD KEEPING

FARNDALE, W.A.J., The Law Relating to Medical Records', *Nursing Times*, July 13, 1978.
GWYNNE, A.L., 'The Legal Importance of Nursing Notes', *Nursing Times*, July 13, 1978.
HOLDECH, R.S., 'The Importance of Patient Care Records', *Nursing Times*, July 13, 1978.

McINTOSH, Jean, 'Getting It Together', *Health and Social Service Journal*, September 30, 1977.

COUNSELLING

BIESTEK, F.P. (1961). *The Casework Relationship*. London: Allen & Unwin.

DAVISON, E.H. (1965). *Social Casework*, London: Baillière Tindall.

De SCHWEINITZ, E. & K. (1962). *Interviewing in the Social Services*, National Council of Social Service.

GARRETT, A. (1942). *Interviewing*. F.S.A.A.

KEITH LUCAS, Alan. (1957). *Some Casework Concepts for the Public Welfare Worker*, Chapel Hill: University of North Carolina Press.

NURSE, G. (1975). *Counselling and the Nurse*. Aylesbury: H.M. & M. Publishers.

CHAPTER 7

The Health Education Role of the District Nurse

HEALTH EDUCATION

Health Education is concerned with human life and survival. It is based upon the assumption that individual behaviour and group norms can affect the quality of life and health. Health education also assumes that, given sufficient knowledge or training, attitudes and behaviour can be changed to ways which current thought and knowledge consider to be most likely to promote and maintain health.

Modern health education has its base in the sanitary reforms which were a response to the conditions created by the industrial revolution and concomitant urbanization. The agglomeration of large population masses in small geographic areas to serve industry, together with the lack of sanitary services heightened the effect of epidemic disease, of squalor and poverty.

The early sanitary reformers used the collection of statistical data as well as the statements of the workers to commissions of enquiry to provoke the interest of the educated public and promote legislation to control environmental conditions.

Gradually policy changes were introduced on a national level to control industrial conditions, housing, food handling and adulteration, and sanitary services. The sanitary reformers were also active at the individual level in promoting services to educate the general public and in particular the poor on the importance of hygiene. One of the major emphases throughout the history of health education has been the instruction of mothers in the care of babies and children in both health and sickness.

The technological advances in industry, although causing such problems as those highlighted above also contributed to health, as for example the provision of cheap, cotton, washable goods replaced woollen garments and cheap, glazed crockery and steel cooking utensils replaced the less easily cleaned articles of previous years. Much progress has taken place until today many of the environmental hazards to health are governed by legislation, and certain government documents emphasize the importance of the prevention of disease rather than the cure.

Some major problems persist and housing shortages, road traffic injuries, chemical and noise pollution of the environment are among them. Changes in population patterns caused by longevity and birth control as well as migration are presenting us with many elderly people, some of whom have no younger member of the family in the vicinity.

Health education changes to meet changing needs. Literacy for the majority of the population and access to the mass media opens ways of reaching many in their homes. There remains however a need for all health care team members to be active in the field of health education.

Since the earliest days of the modern era of District Nursing, Health Education has been seen as one of the major aspects of the work of the trained District Nurse.

The early pioneers referring to the environmental control and organization of the patient's room spoke of 'good nursing order' and, extending patient care to the other care-givers of the family, often expressed concern for the mothers who bore the brunt of the nursing, taking action to ensure short-term relief of those overworked ladies. Education of both patient and family in the skills of nursing, the control of infection and the prevention of avoidable handicap have also been part of the nurse's role through the years and continue to be so. These areas of her work all show the importance of the district nurse in achieving the main aims of health education, the promotion of health and the prevention of ill health. Health has been defined by the World Health Organization (1960) as a 'state of complete physical, mental, and social well-being and not merely the absence of disease or infirmity.' Health education is the means we use to promote that ideal of positive health.

Caplan[1] classified prevention as threefold. Firstly he described primary prevention which involves action to prevent the occurrence of a problem, e.g. immunization, then secondary prevention covering early detection of illness or deviation from the normal which may be cured or controlled, e.g. screening procedures, and thirdly tertiary prevention dealing with containing or alleviating an established condition, e.g. enabling a patient or his family to adjust to incapacity or chronic illness.

The district nurse is clearly involved in all three aspects of prevention but in the home she is usually present because disease or trauma have already occurred and as she assesses the situation she will, with the patient and the relatives, agree a plan of nursing care and the objectives towards which they will be jointly working. It is in this relationship, a one-to-one working relationship, that the most important work of Health Education lies for the district nurse. In promoting health and preventing ill health she will be looking at the totality of patient needs. This will involve consideration of his mental, physical and social well-being as well as the needs of those relatives who provide the greater part of nursing care. The district nurse will be doing this in the light of her understanding of the individual and family needs, her knowledge of broader social and local cultural patterns, expected disease processes and medical intervention, and the availability of statutory and voluntary services.

ONE–TO–ONE TEACHING

EXAMPLE

Perhaps the most important factor in one-to-one teaching is example. The nurse will show the values which underly her nursing practice as she follows the principles of health education together with her consideration of the patient as a valued person in every action. Her appearance expresses her concern for cleanliness. Her listening to the opinion of the patient and family express her view of them as valued people, important in society, and whose views can contribute to effective care and health. Equally when under pressure of work some aspects of care is rushed or neglected for the day she is, by example, showing that these factors are of lesser importance.

Much of health education is involved with changing attitudes, and attitudes are an expression of the underlying beliefs and values of an individual. These beliefs and values usually reflect the beliefs and values of the group with whom the individual identifies himself. Beliefs can be changed by giving new knowledge but values are much more stable and appear to underline the whole pattern of a person's life. If a man has strong economic values which have influenced his attitudes and beliefs throughout life then the occurrence of a disabling illness which effectively removes him from an earning role may produce negative attitudes towards his physical condition that will effectively prevent his progress toward any form of rehabilitation. It might be that identification with a different group could contribute toward changing this value and assist a positive approach to achieving the maximum health now possible to him, or he might through yet another group find a new way of using his abilities which might wholly or in part restore his earning capacity. Many attitudes appear to be easily adapted or changed. This has obvious advantages as one may find evidence in behaviour that attitudes have changed in response to health education. Its disadvantages are also manifest in that the new attitudes shown may as easily change back. In any case no one attitude exists in isolation but is part of an interacting pattern of attitudes relating to many areas of life. These will be linked to an individual's concept of himself, how he wishes to appear to those important to him and what he feels they will think of him if he behaves in certain ways, and the purely utilitarian assessment of worth to the person concerned.

We need then to consider ways of ensuring that any attitude change that occurs in the desired direction remains more or less permanent. We are aware that attitudes have changed because behaviour changes. This is where the example set by the District Nurse is of vital importance. If the patients and relatives are learning from her example then every time the good example is presented the new learning is strengthened or reinforced. You will remember from memorizing such things as the number of days in the months of the year how repetition fixed the pattern in your mind. Now if asked 'How many days have July?' the rhyme recall seems almost automatic. So the daily example set in relation to the promotion of health can produce different behaviour patterns in those who are watching her and working with her in providing nursing or ensuring that caring skills are learned in a way that promotes and maintains health.

Learning from the example of others is called vicarious learning. An example may be found in the work of rehabilitation with a patient suffering a cerebro-vascular attack. The example set by the nurse in appreciating the problems but ensuring that a positive plan of action is set that aims towards achievable goals of recovery can change the attitude of the patient and relatives to the disaster that has affected their lives. This change in attitude will be reinforced by the nurse by the repeated rewards of encouragement and praise and finally the achievement of the small goals set. Her example of care for the patient as a person who can achieve specific goals and her enabling the relatives to contribute to this process are invaluable in promoting physical and mental health and an essential part of rehabilitation.

OPINION LEADERS

The work of several researchers (Krech *et al.*[2]) in the United States of America has shown the importance of the role of opinion leaders in changing attitudes and behaviour. These opinion leaders are seen by the group concerned to be people with authority and knowledge, whose advice is accepted by the community and acted upon. We may infer from this that some of the most effective health education will be achieved where this type of relationship exists. The district nurse may achieve this relationship but it is important to ensure that the health education objectives that she aims to achieve are clearly stated in the nursing care plans so that all the members of the nursing team work towards the same goals. It is also important to ensure that the other members of the Primary Health Care Team who are in contact with the patient are aware and in agreement with the stated objectives. In this way the influence of the opinion leaders from the health team will be uniform and are there-fore more likely to be effective. However in no way does the primary health care team or any individual have the right to exert undue pressure on a patient or his family in order to produce desired ends. As stated above, one of the aims of healthy social life is the functioning of every individual as a valued member of the group; family and community. This must involve the freedom to reject the values and attitudes of others within the limits of personal and community safety.

KNOWLEDGE TRANSMISSION

One-to-one teaching is also achieved by the transmission of knowledge. The District Nurse brings to her practice in the community the know-ledge that she has gained in basic and post-basic training in, for example, normal bodily function and the processes of disease, modes of the spread of infection, the use of drugs and their side effects and individual development and societal needs. This knowledge she adapts to each family and home she visits in the service of health. An example of this will be found in her work with diabetic patients. Her awareness of the physiological effects of the disease process will cause her to advise the patient on the importance of balancing insulin levels and dietary intake and she will discuss further the varying nutritional needs of a diet to maintain health. She will also advise on regular visits to the optician, and where financial constraints occur she will add information about the supplementary benefits system to the advice with regard to adequate footwear.

It should be unnecessary to stress the importance of maintaining levels of knowledge. This will be achieved by continuing education within the profession and by the nurse's own professional reading. The latest research on specific conditions is usually made available by the specialist voluntary organizations as well as in medical journals.

COMMUNICATION IN HEALTH EDUCATION

Part of the skill which needs to be developed in the area of imparting knowledge is the ability to choose the right moment and to ensure that the message communicated is understood, and then to remember the importance of occasional reiteration in some form. Telling a person a fact once may or may not be effective. If I were of normal hearing and teetering on the edge of a cliff a cry of 'A rope to your right hand' would probably be sufficient as fear would have focussed my attention. Too much fear though might cause me to forget which is my right hand.

Many studies have looked at the effect of fear in producing a response and the results seem to be conflicting. It would seem that response follows a U-shaped curve with certain levels of fear arousal being required to initiate a response, but very high levels of fear causing a rejection or defence reaction from the cause of fear. This is important when communicating information to our patients. Many of our patients and their families are anxious and some are frightened and this can be an effective block to communication. There is a need to listen to the very real fears and anxieties that may be expressed and false reassurance is no comfort. The nurse who is giving an impression of overwork will fail here. She may well be rushed, but part of her professional approach must be to appear unhurried and there is a need to organize her caseload to enable patients to discuss their concerns. Having been permitted this expression of anxiety the patient may then be in a condition to hear the message being conveyed.

Another equally important aspect of allowing time to listen is the need to find out the existing level of knowledge and understanding. Some patients will have read widely on the subject of their condition, already belong to a voluntary action group and stand in need of no further teaching on the subject. Once this fact is decided the nurse will then only need to check that appropriate health maintaining and promoting behaviour is taking place, and to share with this patient new research findings and information as it becomes available. Teaching needs to start where the patient and relatives are in understanding both of the diagnosis of the condition, and within the context of the patient's environment. The particular skill of teaching is in building bridges that link knowledge already possessed and permit a person to reach out to new levels of knowledge. Obviously to continue the analogy, the bridge must have firm foundations in already extant and accurate knowledge.

Listening as well as observing plays its part in finding out whether the communication has been understood. On this evaluation it may be necessary to re-think the educational aims involved. The elderly patient may well have understood the explanation given by the nurse, the doctor and the hospital about taking a high bran diet but may have preferred white bread through over eighty years of life. Further telling will only produce a twinkle in the eye and appreciation of their concern. What alternative ways might there be of balancing the bran intake? Perhaps another elderly person who has had to face the same difficulty and has overcome it might be a better motivation to changed dietary habits. Other factors to consider would also be finance, availability of high bran products and slightly different recipes.

DISCUSSION

This leads us to another aspect of one-to-one teaching, namely discussion. Education has often been seen in the past to be the passing on of facts. A patient has been told and therefore he knows. We suggested earlier that one of the particular skills of teaching is to build bridges that enable people to reach out to new things. Discussion is particularly valuable here as the combined thoughts of patient, relative and nurse are expressed and looked at from different angles with each contributing problems and solutions. Having produced possible courses of action in this way then the nurse, patient and relations are more likely to work together to achieve a positive result. The best aims and solutions come from the patient and his relative as they are more likely to have a personal commitment to achieving them.

TEACHING PRACTICAL SKILLS

District nurses are also, as part of their teaching role, required to pass on practical skills. One of the difficulties that can arise from the very skill the nurse possesses is the tendency to try to teach too much at one time. For example, when lifting a heavy, incapacitated person alone the skilled nurse is automatically considering patient posture, comfort and safety, the factors affecting pressure areas such as wrinkles in clothing and sheets, pillow edges and adequate support, while also considering the principles of lifting and those factors affecting her own health.

Where do you start when passing on this skill to the relatives, as it is a very positive aspect of health education concerned with:

1. The prevention of pressure sores and the pain which results from bad posture, in the patient.
2. The prevention of physical strain or damage in the relatives.

Start with the patient. What do we wish to achieve? Then to the relative. What do they know and what do they need to know initially? Then to the teaching. Can you break it down into small, easily achieved steps that can be clearly explained? Can you and the patient and the relative work together on this? However all the telling and showing in the world will not pass on a practical skill. Such skills are achieved by practice, at first with help, then under advice and finally alone. Where possible of course one would try to avoid lifting very heavy patients alone and ensure as soon as possible the provision of mechanical aids.

GROUP TEACHING

With the move towards the provision of primary health care through teams of staff based on general practice populations there has developed an increasing involvement in small group teaching for the district nurse. Groups of people with a common concern, for example overweight, stoma, diabetes mellitus or coronary heart disease are being formed with the aim of working together to achieve a greater understanding of their physical condition, ameliorating side effects and learning how to live a normal life within the bounds of their special problems.

CONTENT OF TEACHING

Taking part in small group teaching can be very worrying for many and it is potentially more difficult than giving a straight lecture, on a topic on which you are an expert, to a large group. There one may shelter behind the security of the lectern and the lecture notes, whereas in the small group there is the expectation of group involvement and the give and take of discussion.

Most people when asked to participate in small group sessions commence a frantic search for information on every aspect of the subject at hand. A fairly good starting point, as there is nothing like the assurance of mastery of the subject for bolstering confidence when facing a group. The search for accurate information should include the latest material available and it is necessary to assess the value of what is read. On what are the statements based?

The following questions need to be asked. Are they the result of research and was the sample of a large enough size to be able to generalize from the results? Is it opinion and how expert was the person giving the opinion? Is it written with a deliberate bias to make a point or an unconscious bias because of the emotional or professional involvement of the author? When was it written? Is it out of date? Evaluate what is read, analyse and make your own conclusions. It is worthwhile to be thorough and organized in gathering information. If you intend to quote ensure that you give credit to the author, having available the author's name, date of publication as well as the title of the work and the publisher, as some member of the group may be interested enough to want to read further. Quite a good idea is to use postcards with the quote written out in full and the source of origin at the bottom, this can then be filed for future reference. Small box files are fairly cheap or one can be made out of a shoe-box. Having gathered the material there is a need for a shift in the focus of your thinking. Obviously you cannot stand before a group and pass on to them all this wonderful wealth of knowledge you have acquired. It might be unsuitable, it would probably be unnecessary.

SELECTION OF MATERIAL

Turn your mind to the group to be taught. Consider the reason for their forming part of this group and what you think they are coming for. They will have between them a lot of knowledge already, certainly practical knowledge of how it feels, and some of the problems as well as folklore contributed by friends and relatives. Many will have read about their condition and they will have discussed it with medical and possibly other nursing staff. Why have they asked you to take a session, and what is your particular contribution and expertise? Where do you fit in to the whole and what aspects are other people dealing with? This should narrow down somewhat the great store of knowledge that you have available. So consider again what do you want to do in the time available. What is really important in your opinion for this group of people and, given the limitations of time, how much do you think it is feasible to include in the session under consideration? Are there other ways of imparting some of the crucial facts? Perhaps if the groups are very interested, a clear handout giving some essential information could be made available to them. Not an overcrowded, closely typed page but an easily read one, a well-spaced brief statement of some facts that you think would be of use to them for reference. It is possible that some society or group has already produced an attractive handout that covers the information you wish to give in this way. Your colleagues, the specialist voluntary society or your local health education officer may be able to help you in this respect.

Having collected your information and concluded the needs of the group your next step is to decide your objectives for the session. It might be helpful to think of the end of the session and state your intention in some form such as: At the end of the session the group will be able to state or list certain things or will have discussed the pros and cons of certain forms of behaviour. The statement of short-term objectives in this way enables one to focus the attention onto what it is possible to achieve in the time available and then to consider the best way to achieve it.

For example, if you wish a group to work together on changing their dietary habits it will be necessary to gain consensus on what they hope to achieve. Merely telling them a list of do's and don'ts is unlikely to persuade a group of people to work together and provide group support for each other in pursuit of a common aim. If they are given the opportunity to discuss the needs for a changed diet, to express their doubts and eventually to make a commitment, then to come back after a short trial to discuss successes and failures and renew their commitment, a change in dietary habits is more likely to take place.

Therefore decide on your objectives and choose the method of teaching that is most likely to be successful. If you wish certain facts to be recalled you will select a method that reiterates these facts vocally and visually in order to facilitate their recall. You may state a point, illustrate it in some way, write it down, use a picture or story, ask the group to comment on it. Summarize at the end the points made and this way ensure that important facts are salient in the session. Be clear in your own mind so that you may present the information logically. If you intend to use visual aids remember that visually presented material is often more clearly recalled than verbally presented material, so resist the temptation to illustrate unimportant details in this way, just because you have a good visual aid, as these might well crowd out the more important points that are really basic to your session. You are now ready to start preparing your teaching plan. The subject has been researched and the knowledge is up-to-date and factually correct. The group knowledge and needs have been considered. The objectives are set and the most suitable teaching methods considered.

PLANNING THE PRESENTATION

It is again necessary to be logical in that a session should have a beginning, a middle and an end. The beginning is to set the scene, capture the imagination of the group, to state intent. The end is to summarize where you have been, to pick up the most important areas that have been considered. The middle is the bulk of the session and can well be divided into different sections that flow logically each from the other. If you wish to divide the sections more clearly you may summarize the discussion that has taken place and by a question or statement lead the group on to another point or section that you wish to consider. As you prepare your notes for a session it is good to have the sections clearly indicated and have some statement of the amount of time you might spend discussing certain aspects. You will find with experience that the more you involve the group in discussion the less ground will be covered. This makes the selection and planning of content even more important. If discussion is however achieving the objectives it is better to cover a small amount of material thoroughly, to the satisfaction of the group, and return another time to the rest. In general people enjoy a session in which they have been able to take part in a constructive way.

GROUP CONTROL

One of the skills you will develop as you use discussion methods of teaching will be group control, enabling the shy person to speak and controlling the group member who tries to take over or to lead the discussion off the subject. Each group member needs to feel that his participation is valuable. Smiling and eye contact are part of the skills of eliciting comment and encouraging more comment as are nodding and grunting (appropriately). A short agreement and the removal of eye contact from someone who is monopolizing the conversation is sometimes effective in allowing another to speak.

GROUP LEADERSHIP

Your role as the leader of the discussion is to ensure that it keeps reasonably to the subject, to feed in accurate information, to ensure that everyone has a chance to participate by encouraging the shy, controlling the dominant participant and then to draw the conclusion at the end. Many inexperienced group leaders find a brief silence difficult to live with and anxieties as to their leadership role make the brief silence seem an endless void. This causes them to rush into speech often to the exclusion of a member who was about to participate. Short silences can be quite comfortable and useful in allowing people to think or decide how to contribute.

Roles in groups are rarely static as groups have dynamic patterns of relationships. As the leader it is necessary to exercise leadership and the authority of leadership without dominating and yet not so inadequately that the leadership is ignored and the views expressed rejected or the leadership passes entirely to a member of the group. If a group is very passive it may be necessary to take an opposing view in order to enable the group to think more widely round the subject. This role can be called devil's advocate. It is possible that a member of the group may act in this way.

Where deeply divided issues arise the leader may need to act as chairman balancing the views and possibly not voicing his own opinion in a way that might alienate half the group and effectively stop any reasoned discussion or learning for them.

If the preparation has been thorough it is most likely that you may be seen as an authoritative consultant who is able to feed in knowledge to fuel discussion. Often of course this will be your initial role as you commence the session with some positive input to act as a basis for discussion.

TEACHING NOTES

Your notes for a discussion will probably be something like the following form. On an outside cover the subject, the group, the time available, a statement of objectives and the way you aim to achieve them, a teaching method, and for your own future reference a bibliography of sources that you used in preparing the session. Inside will be your introduction, the discussion of your session and points you intend to summarize in conclusion. Your notes should be brief as reminders of the topics you intend to introduce. If you write out in full every word you intend to say there may be the temptation to read the notes which is extremely boring. In fact it would probably be more effective to hand the written essay to the group and to read and to spend time discussing any points they would like elucidated. One way of preparing teaching notes is outlined below:

Table 5. A method of preparing teaching notes

Outline	Content	Time	Method	Visual Aids
Introduction	Quotes			
	Details	5 mins	Tell	
Point 1	Details	10 mins	Ask, tell and discuss	Flannel graph
Point 2	Details	10 mins	Ask, tell and discuss	Flannel graph
Point 3	Details	10 mins	Discuss	Handout
Conclusion	Summary	5 mins	Tell	

You would also need a plan of how you intend to organize the material on your flannel graph or, if you are using a blackboard or overhead projector, exactly how and what you might write down. You can probably recall sessions that you have attended in the past where the writing was illegible and muddled and looked as though it had been written by a tipsy spider as it staggered up and down the board. The information you write down is a visual aid to reinforce the important facts that you wish to be remembered from the session. It is also available for reference when you summarize at the end of the session.

One of the advantages you will find from working with small groups is that the rapport you establish with the group and the verbal interaction that takes place during sessions will increase your understanding of individual and group needs. As your skills as a group leader create a comfortable environment you will learn a great deal from the groups and about the groups. This means that you can assess during the session if an individual has special needs that might be helped by you or another member of the Primary Health Care Team. This rapport also gives you feedback as to how far any particular session may go and whether the pace at which you are proceeding is appropriate.

EVALUATION

At the end of the teaching session comes one of the most important parts of the process – evaluation. As with nursing care there is the need to look at what has been done and assess it with a view to considering future needs and planning further programmes. Evaluate as objectively as you can what happened in the session and why it happened in that way. Note the things that might be developed on a future occasion.

Finally, always take a fresh look if you are asked to repeat the session to another group. A sage said that you can never step into the same river twice because the water has flowed on. A session that was a dream of perfection once will be different next time. You are different, more confident with success, further away from your thinking and planning. New research may have been published. The group is different, new people, different personalities, new feelings. Take a fresh look at the topic, the group and the session in order to meet the new situation.

REFERENCES

1. CAPLAN, G. (1961). An approach to Community Mental Health. London: Tavistock.
2. KRECH, D., CRUTCHFIELD, R.S. & BALLACHEY, E.L. (1962). *Individuals in Society*. New York: McGraw-Hill.

FURTHER READING

Small Group Teaching (1976). A report by the Group for Research and Innovation in Higher Education. The Nuffield Foundation.

RUNSWICK, H. & DAVIS, C.C. (1976). *Health Education: practical teaching techniques*. H.M. & M. Publishers Ltd.

WARREN, N. & JAHODA, M. (1973). *Attitudes*. Harmondsworth: Penguin.

Prevention and Health: everybody's business. (1976). London: HMSO.

SUTHERLAND, I. (1979). *Health Education: Perspectives and Choices*. London: George Allen & Unwin.

IRWIN, V. & SPIRA, M. (1977). *Basic Health Education*. London: Longman.

SECTION TWO

The Health and Social Context

CHAPTER 8

The National Health Service

STRUCTURE

It has been difficult for anybody to write about the structure of the National Health Service during the seventies. Before 1974 there was the mounting uncertainty of what reorganization would entail. After 1974 difficulties arose from the problems of implementing the reforms of the reorganization.[1] The 1980s it would appear are to be little different. A Royal Warrant was issued on the 19 May, 1976 setting up a Royal Commission on the National Health Service under the chairmanship of Sir Alexander Merrison. The Commission issued its report in July 1979 (Merrison Report).[2] The report recommended some quite wide ranging changes to the structure and operation of the health service. Uncertainty now arises about the extent and manner of any implementation that may result. As the seventies drew to a close the government issued a consultative paper on the National Health Service in England and Wales entitled *Patients First*.[3] The government required comments on it to be completed by the end of April.

In August, *The Health Service Act, 1980*[4] received the Royal Assent. It is envisaged that the ensuing structural changes will be effected by the end of 1983. It should be noted that the legislation discussed relates only to England and Wales, it is different in Scotland where there is separate legislation.

In case anyone should hope that the dust might then comfortably settle, the appropriate Secretaries of State warn that the pattern proposed '. . . must not be seen as a final and rigid blueprint to last for all time. On the contrary it will fail if it does not embody within itself the ability to respond flexibly and positively to the future needs of the people.[5] The paper does not, however, particularly relish the prospect of further change. The approach it favours is that to which administrators refer as incremental change or a little at a time. Its virtue is recommended in the Latin motto *Festina lente* or 'Make haste slowly'. This, it is hoped, will permit change that can be adequately digested, but some may worry that the portions may be too small to sustain life.

While it might be laudable to follow the example of the consultative paper's title and put patients first in the following account of the National Health Service structure, it might be considered by many a little too idealistic. This summary will therefore follow a fairly well-established tradition and begin nearer the top of the administrative hierarchy.

THE SECRETARY OF STATE

At the summit is the Secretary of State. He of course is a government minister and responsible to Parliament for 'the promotion in England and Wales of a comprehensive health service designed to secure improvement:

1. In the physical and mental health of the people of those countries.
2. In the prevention, diagnosis and treatment of illness, and for that purpose to provide or secure the effective provision of services. . . .'[6]

He will be influenced in how he promotes or restricts the service by parliamentary debates, by the general economic and political climate, by the priorities and values of his particular political orientation, by expert advisory committees and by specific health interest groups. He is also advised by his civil servants at the Department of Health and Social Security (DHSS). Like other ministers he is regularly required to account to Parliament in debates and at question time and various committees may seek a response from him. He is assisted in this work by his junior ministers and under some governments by a political adviser. He is not accountable for the clinical decisions of the medical profession within the service.

THE DEPARTMENT OF HEALTH AND SOCIAL SECURITY (DHSS)

The civil service department which the Secretary of State heads is the Department of Health and Social Security, formed by a merger of the Ministries of Health and of Social Security in 1968. The chief civil servant at the DHSS is a Permanent Secretary who is responsible for all monies spent in the service. He may be called to account by the Comptroller and Auditor-General as well as by certain committees of the House of Commons.

The DHSS is monitored by the Treasury and its budget proposals are achieved in negotiation with Treasury representatives before being put to the Cabinet by the Secretary of State.

The DHSS organizes its personnel about certain major objectives. These concern, support for the Secretary of State in providing central leadership within the Service, helping the Secretary of State to decide priorities and standards at national level, assisting the Secretary of State in advising the appropriate subsidiary levels of national priorities, helping to negotiate satisfactory pay and conditions of service for NHS personnel, undertaking negotiations with the Treasury and Civil Service Department and finally it provides support for financial management. The Merrison report favoured devolving more financial responsibility to Regional authorities[7] but government preference appears to be to leave things as they are.

THE REGIONAL HEALTH AUTHORITY (RHA)

The RHA acts as a link between the DHSS and the more localized units of the health service. Under the 1974 reorganization there were the Area Health Authorities (AHAs). The consultative paper *Patients First* suggests, as did the Merrison Report, that in the future the Area Health Authority will be replaced by a District Health Authority (DHA). This is in fact what 'the 1980 Act' now requires.

The RHA also has responsibility for distributing resources according to national requirements. It is thus concerned with major building projects, the development of medical specialties and the implementation of monitoring of strategic plans.

The strong monitoring role given to the RHA under the 1974 reorganization may the consultative paper suggests be modified. Some of the monitoring of district management and service development could at some future date be entrusted to an advisory group of NHS officers reporting to a DHA.[8]

Some non-clinical support services may be made more responsive to district level budgetting by introducing some kind of fee for service arrangement.

Finally, the RHA has an important role in formulating, from information and developments in the field, advice which will serve '. . . to assist the Secretary of State to establish realistic national policies and priorities.'[9]

THE RISE AND DECLINE OF THE AREA HEALTH AUTHORITY (AHA)

In the various proposals prior to the 1974 reorganization there had been a stage at which the AHAs were envisaged as being directly responsible to the Secretary of State and Regional Health Councils were seen as advisory bodies to the AHA.[10] Subsequently the then Secretary of State, Sir Keith Joseph, sought to establish a clear managerial chain of command, with the AHA subordinate to the RHA and the RHA subordinate to the DHSS. The strong managerial function was reflected in the emphasis on appointments being made on a managerial rather than a representative basis. This latter emphasis reappears in the consultative paper *Patients First*.

The 1974 reorganization made the AHA the lowest tier of statutory responsibility. It was responsible for ensuring that comprehensive health services were provided to all in the area who needed them. In relation to its population it was also responsible for planning services, establishing priorities and allocating resources. These requirements it might implement through its constituent districts.

The Merrison Report found that in representations made to it, the AHA tier was the one most frequently criticized. The report recognized the need to simplify decision making and communications and the necessity of improving coordination. It further appreciated the duplication that arose between the area and district administration. The report was also dubious about the extent to which collaboration had been achieved by making area boundaries coterminous with those of local authorities. The report therefore recommended that beneficial simplicity could be achieved by abolishing the area level.

This view found support in the consultative paper *Patients First* which emphasised the need to delegate more responsibility downwards to the front line of hospital and consumer services. In the House of Commons Mr Patrick Jenkins, the Secretary of State, stated that the main thrust of the government proposals was . . . 'to push responsibility down to hospital and primary Service care levels'.[11]

Hence the stage was set for the AHAs to be replaced by new statutory District Health Authorities (DHAs), this was done by 'the 1980 Act'.

DISTRICTS IN THE ASCENDANCY

The 1974 reorganization proposals saw the district as the basic operational unit for providing integrated health care. The 'grey book' defined the district as '. . . a population served by community health services supported by the specialist services of a district general hospital'.[12]

The number of districts within an AHA varied. Each district was intended to reflect a 'natural health care district'. This envisaged a population of about 250 000. This population would typically comprise 60 000 children of whom 500 might be physically handicapped and 200 mentally handicapped. There would be upwards of 35 000 people over sixty five. Of this latter group 4500 might be physically handicapped, 800 in hospital, 800 in old people's homes and 1000 might be alone and in need of domiciliary care. This population would be covered by about five social work area teams and ten primary care teams.

The attainment of such an 'ideal' district might be difficult to achieve and the 1979 consultative paper acknowledged that the district pattern might have to be modified to accommodate various local features. These features are settlement and transport patterns and well-established community identities. It should also reflect what it called 'the catchment areas of major hospitals'. It should be big enough to support the range of services associated with a district general hospital but be small enough for personnel not to experience the authority as remote. Finally, some coterminous boundaries should be established perhaps involving districts combining to match social service or education authority boundaries.[13]

The district of the eighties, known individually as, for example, the Udchurch Health Authority, is a statutory health authority replacing the AHA and subordinate to the RHA. It will be responsible for planning, development and management within the guidelines set by the RHA.

DHAs in consultation with their regions will decide how to divide or maintain various services previously provided by the AHA such as the ambulance service.

FAMILY PRACTITIONER COMMITTEES (FPCs)

The 1974 reorganization of the NHS required AHAs to set up Family Practitioner Committees. These administered GPs' contracts, negotiated disputes and listed the GPs engaged by the authority. The AHA consulted the FPC in planning and organizing family practitioner services including the development of health centres and schemes for attaching nurses to general practice.

The Merrison report proposed that these FPCs should be abolished along with the AHAs. It argued that the existence of FPCs meant that there was a partially independent sector which posed problems of coordination, collaboration and integrated planning. If the new DHAs assume responsibility from the FPCs they could be more effective in positively influencing the distribution and quality of practice premises and the proper coordination of hospital and community care.[14] The government proposals in *Patients First* however saw no advantage here and presumably were aware of the reluctance of the medical profession to lose them. As 'the 1980 Act' makes clear, the FPCs will stay and, if necessary, cover more than one district. This would seem to go against the principles of administrative simplification advocated in the consultative document.

POLICY

Professor Titmuss in his book *Social Policy*[15] points out that policy is necessary where questions of choice arise. There is no point in having a policy on the weather since there is nothing anybody can do about it. Health and illness can to some extent be influenced, and choices have therefore to be made. Who makes the choices and why, is the basis of policy which can hardly be anything other than controversial and hence in some sense political. All that can be attempted in the limited scope of this chapter, is to illustrate something of the scope of health service policy.

MARKET PROVISION

The need to curtail public expenditure and hence to contain public expectations leads some to question the basic principle that the major part of health service provision should be free at the point of delivery. Some would increase the range of services for which charges are made. Others argue that choice should be extended so that the patient could be more selective in the level and conditions of treatment, with more privacy and more personal attention. This, it is argued, could be achieved by considerably extending the private sector and increasing funding through voluntary insurance schemes and direct payment. The basic health facilities could be covered by a voucher scheme or a means-tested, tax-credit scheme.

The arguments against these proposals generally develop the idea that where health facilities are provided on the basis of the ability to pay, the better provision will inevitably be drawn towards those with the money, rather than those with the greatest need. Nor, of course, is it guaranteed to eliminate waste. It is difficult for people rendered anxious about their own or their family's health, to resist the glossy advertisement. Professional ethics are no guarantee against pushing up the price for trimmings and over elaborate diagnostic procedures, according to what the market will bear, rather than what is needed.

Within the NHS, it is argued expenditure might be better saved by more effectively controlling drug production and prescribing, and monitoring many clinical procedures. Cochrane in his book *Effectiveness and efficiency in the National Health Service*[16] made a strong case for introducing random controlled trials to reduce the incidence of treatments which cannot be demonstrated to be effecttive. This of course runs up against the difficulty of persuading the medical profession, or any other profession for that matter, to subject its clinical judgement to scrutiny.

PRIORITIES

A more radical policy question directed towards priorities in the National Health Service is posed by Professor McKeown.[17] He demonstrates, in a well-supported case, that the major improvements in health care are primarily attributable to nutritional advances. The second significant factor he identifies as progressive developments in hygiene, especially in water and sewage control and food hygiene. He points out that if one considers the historical evidence, a whole range of major diseases were declining before chemotherapeutic techniques were introduced. Indeed chemotherapy was frequently introduced only at the tail end of a decline. This is well illustrated by the major decline in respiratory tuberculosis between the years 1838 and 1948. While streptomycin has reduced the number of deaths by 51% in the period since its introduction, its total contribution to the reduction of mortality from the disease, since cause of death was first recorded, is only 3.2%. McKeown points out that crisis-oriented clinical medicine would seem these days to require a lower priority than care and preventive medicine. Yet the reverse seems to be the case, with care in the less prestigious fields of geriatric and mental incapacity receiving a relatively lower share of resources.

RAWP

A third policy area which has received attention recently is redistribution, and the attempt to redistribute resources more equitably between the regions in the National Health Service in England and Wales. The case for this was fully propounded in the report of the Resource Allocation Working Party (RAWP).[18] It recommended that regions, which had consistently received more in relation to their needs than other regions, should have their finances restrained while allocations to underprovided regions should be increased, so that eventually 'there would be equal opportunity of access to health care for people at equal risk'.[19]

Considerable resistance was generated by those who were in regions destined to experience constraints. Controversy focussed on the measures used to identify need. The working party judged that the actual death rate in a region compared with the expected death rate would indicate the greater or lesser rate of illness. The formula used was complicated by the need to take into account the age, sex and distribution of the population. It was also difficult to assess the resources of a region. There was, therefore, room to question the reliability of the formula. The press finding bad news more newsworthy than good news concentrated on the cuts rather than the benefits. Prestigious professionals were more aggravated as the adjustments came on top of modifications intended to give greater priority to particular disadvantaged groups. Nevertheless, the government tentatively embarked on the proposals having moderated the impact by extending the time scale. However, with a change of government and severe expenditure cuts any significant effect is now hardly discernible. Despite this, the problems and principles remain to challenge future policies.

Groups will have different interests, allegiances, aims and priorities, there are therefore important areas of choice and principle and hence of controversy. The social and economic and political context in which these choices have to be made are themselves subject to change and negotiation. The National Health Service itself is an arrangement dependent for its maintenance, improvement or erosion, on the aims, strategies and activities of different groups both internal and external to it. It would seem difficult for the district nurse interested in the home care of her patients to be anything but concerned and involved in achieving a satisfactory outcome of the policy choices involved in the National Health Service.

PLANNING

If policy choices are to be implemented then plans have to be drawn up and financed. Within the National Health Service there is a planning cycle intended to achieve this. It is meant to integrate and coordinate the plans of all levels of the Service.

Each statutory tier of the National Health Service administration maintains a strategic plan which offers a long-term framework covering the aims of the service for between ten and fifteen years ahead. It also provides a programme within which short-term operations are planned. The strategic framework is revised every three years and modified to accord with any changes in current provision.

The short term or operational planning cycle can be seen as beginning when the DHSS receives the regional annual planning reports. The DHSS then takes these into account in devising its own plans in consultation with the regions. The DHSS are then in a position to issue planning guidelines to the RHAs along with information on the availability of the necessary finance. The DHAs will work to a similar programme. The implications are considered in consultation with the appropriate Community Health Councils (CHCs), advisory committees and relevant local authorities. The DHAs will dovetail their planning with the RHA so that the RHA is fully informed when it draws up regional plans. Thus there are two current flows. One channels guidance, information and resources down from the DHSS to the regions and districts. The other is a reciprocal flow of information, modifications, changes, progress and plans, directed upwards from the DHA to the RHA and DHSS.

This system affords vital channels of communications. The government consultative paper *Patients First* accepted the general advantages of the current planning process but hoped that the excision of the area tier and statutory strengthening of the district would provide a more direct, sensitive and efficient tool. The Secretary of State addressing the House of Commons expressed the belief that 'the closer management decisions are taken to the point of patients care the more likely it is that patients' interests will predominate'.[20] This weighting of the planning process towards the District level should mean that the District Nurse practitioners' voice should have a better chance of being registered through her District Nursing Officer, with a significant and effective planning team. With the abolition of the AHAs it is to be expected that the planning procedures will shortly be reviewed.

RELATIONS IN THE NATIONAL HEALTH SERVICE

The relations that exist in the National Health Service are manifold and complex. Relations exist between the National Health Service and other departments. There are relations with central and local government. There are relations both external and internal with professional associations, trade unions and various voluntary bodies. The different tiers of management involve relations between personnel and administrative groups. The different branches of the service also have to establish working relations. Any attempt to cover all of these in less than a complete book would be futile. In this section attention will simply be drawn to some of the problems that arise in some working relations which affect the operation of the service.

MANAGEMENT TEAMS

The National Health Service reorganization emphasized in its arrangements the need to integrate the contribution of different sectors. It also considered that if decisions were to be effectively implemented they should have the support of all the sectors involved. The method of achieving this was to relate the different sectors by establishing teams. Thus at each level of the service are to be found a series of teams. At District level the District Management Team comprises the District Administrator, the District Finance Officer, the District Nursing Officer, the District Community Physician and the Chairman and Vice-Chairman of the District Medical Committee. As a team they are responsible to the District Health Authority, though the individual members are accountable for their individual sectors, except of course the Medical Committee members who are representatives.

The District Health Authorities collaborate with Local Authorities through Joint Consultative Committees. Where a local authority contains two DHAs there need be only one committee covering both DHAs.[21] The Family Practitioners' Committee is a statutory committee and under 'the 1980 Act' will be linked to one or more District Health Authorities. Finally, the Health Authorities are supported by Professional Advisory Committees.

This structure is replicated at Regional level with a Regional Team of Officers and Professional Advisory Committees supporting the Regional Health Authority.

Decision making

Several difficulties have been experienced with the relations in teams and decision-making by team consensus when the decision must be a unanimous one. One difficulty is that reaching total agreement can be a slow and painful business, thus decisions can be seriously delayed. They can be even slower if the teams cannot agree and the decision is passed to a superior, if no speedier, team. The presence of a team may also make individual members unwilling to take decisions in their own area of concern for fear of offending team colleagues. Thus decisions tend to be pushed upwards to the team above which caused further delays and generates staff frustrations. Again members may try to keep controversial issues off the agenda because of the interminable and indecisive debates that consensus team management may encourage. Alternatively difficult decisions may be passed upwards. Clashes of temperament or the dominance of some members can exacerbate delays.

These difficulties suggest two possible modifications. The first is to shorten the lines of communication and to reduce the levels for referral. This is the intention behind the abolition of the Area Health Authority. The result of this is not only to shorten lines of communication and reduce a tier, but the inevitably more remote relationship between a District Health Authority and a Regional Health Authority should discourage unnecessary referral upwards.

A second modification would be to strengthen the line management. This could involve selecting the team personnel on the basis of expertise and special function as well as proven ability, installing a chief executive and at the same time removing the necessity for consensus decisions. In a structure like the National Health Service with contending and powerful groups this move would be fraught with difficulties and might involve greater costs than the delays of consensus management by corporate teams. The 1980 Act while expecting consensus, weakens it somewhat by saying that it does not mean unanimity at all costs. It requires that significant differences of view should be reported to the authority.

RELATIONS WITH LOCAL AUTHORITIES

Relations between the National Health Service and the Local Authorities are another source of difficulty. It is hoped that good relations may be facilitated by making District Health Authority boundaries coterminous with those of the social services or education authority. This is an important relationship since the integration of many services require coordination between those supplied by the Local Authority and those supplied by the National Health Service. It is, for example, unsatisfactory if patients ready for discharge find that community resources cannot be readily made available for satisfactory continuity in care. As well as coterminous boundaries local authority members are appointed to the health authorities. Health authorities provide staff for environmental health and personal social functions while local authorities may make social work staff available to health centres. There are also the Joint Consultative Committees for the two authorities in England and Wales. Finally, joint funding exists for certain projects of common interest.

Difficulties nevertheless arise since joint authorities can result in neither accepting responsibility. Coordination of services may also be difficult because divergencies arise in agreeing priorities. Public expenditure cuts may restrict one side more than the other so the local authority may be reluctant to engage in expenditure which it may hope the health authority may otherwise bear. Equally they may be reluctant to support jointly-funded projects if they may have to provide full funding after six years. Projects in the health sector compete for finance with other sectors for which local authorities are responsible. The local authority is also subject to political pressures as well as budget pressures from ratepayers and voters. Thus collaboration involves more complex issues than simply setting up the joint team.

It has been suggested that these difficulties might be eased if client groups could be transferred so that they become the sole responsibility of one authority or the other. Here the difficulty might be to transfer the staff. If, for example, personal Social Services were brought under the National Health Service coordination might be improved. Health personnel might favour this but it is likely that the social work profession would oppose it.

This leads to a more radical suggestion that the National Health Service, like the Education Service should be operated by the Local Authority. This would reduce many of the problems referred to in this section. It would eliminate problems of divided responsibility and facilitate integrated planning. Community Health Councils would not be necessary since the local authority can be said to represent the consumer. Sensitivity to local needs might be increased though national standards might be more difficult to achieve. The medical profession has long resisted such a move and is hardly likely to respond with favour now. The Merrison Report while recommending no such changes does foresee possible developments in this direction if at some future date there should be some form of regional government.[22]

RELATIONS BETWEEN OCCUPATIONAL GROUPS

Relations between health service personnel have tended to become more sensitive. The doctors with a tradition of independence and an ethic of optimal care for their patient find the constraints of a large organizational structure irksome. Nor are the doctors generally very partial to what they may see as the political voice of the lay representative. They may also feel that the more traditional unquestioned status and authority of the doctor is increasingly challenged as other occupational groups are strengthened.

Administrators with an undoubtedly difficult task in rather new circumstances find themselves the scapegoats for every difficulty in the service. They have to achieve and implement programmes in the face of sometimes dubious team decisions and against very independent-minded professionals over whom they may have little influence. The administrator may find the cumulative financial consequences of some clinical decisions formidable yet be in no position to challenge them.

Larger organizational structures and increasing technology have led to significant new staff groupings and greater accessibility for unionizing endeavours. It has also meant that more key activities have arisen influencing wide areas making them vulnerable to threats of industrial action. The familial groupings and loyalties of the smaller units that existed in earlier days have tended to be eroded in the large, increasingly remote structures of the health service. Pay negotiating structures become more complex and pay differentials achieve higher visibility and multiply. An unwillingness to pay substantial rises to the very numerous low-paid groups because of the overall expense, as well as the breakdown of delicate balances between other groups, exacerbated by pay policies has led to outbreaks of various forms of 'industrial action' among doctors as well as ancillary staff. The effects of these can sour relations for much longer than the period of crisis action.

Attempts have been made to improve some of these difficulties in personnel relations in the area of the clinical task by the idea of 'multidisciplinary clinical teams'. Difficulties arise here over questions of leadership as the Merrison Report indicates.[23] In its evidence to the Royal Commission the Royal College of Nursing suggested that 'the leadership role should be determined by the situation'.[24] The problem then arises as to who should evaluate the situation.

Perhaps the effect of shifting responsibility downwards to district level may lead to a closer identification of personnel with their district and patients and promote the re-establishment of trust and loyalty between members. Certainly the future would seem to be one where more negotiation has to be undertaken and more flexible structures devised.

RELATIONS IN THE PRIMARY HEALTH CARE TEAM

District nurses may be more familiar with the problems of operating relations in a Primary Health Care Team. Here the assumption is that they try to work as a team and not as isolated individuals. As in the hospital the idea of the team was to integrate the care delivered to the patient by different professional groups. In an article entitled 'Teamwork in theory and practice',[25] McIntosh and Dingwall study some of the barriers to team work which they found in a primary health care setting. They suggest that authority relations set in the hospital training setting may not be disturbed in the primary care setting, whereas the more critical training of the Health Visitor and her own referral sources may make her more independent minded and more challenging to the doctor and district nurse. She may be further isolated by the uncertain perception that the district nurse and doctor may have about her role. The male doctor on the other hand with his traditional, proprietorial position, his traditional status, legal responsibility, not to mention his susceptibilities to dominate, may not be very willing to participate in a very flexible way in a cooperative team. As Stein points out in *The Doctor-Nurse Game*[26] the nurse has to engage in Machiavellian plots and strategies to persuade the doctor that her suggestion ought to be heeded. Anciliary Staff and patients may reflect the hierarchical traditional view of Doctor and Nurse, making the development of initiatives by the nurse difficult. As the district nurse is well aware and as Graham Woods points out 'It is all too easy to assume that simply putting a group of professionals together in appropriately equipped premises will create a satisfactory working team.'[27] Further difficulties arise in integrating the delivery of the nursing and medical provision with those of Welfare. Attempts to improve this by arranging some coterminosity in the training of Social Workers and some health service personnel run up against barriers of different professional orientations and practice ethos, not to mention the practical difficulties of coordinating groups on courses of different lengths. In some areas locating social work offices in or alongside health centres has met with a measure of success although it is by no means guaranteed.

The difficulties might tempt some to abandon the attempt to improve relations. Yet this would be to fail the patient whose life is made more stressful and uncertain where they are subject to the vagaries of uncoordinated provision.

THE DELIVERY OF HOME CARE

In the context of the discussion that follows, home care will be taken to mean the provision of health care for the individual resident at home, as opposed to someone for whom care is provided in an institutional setting.

The provision of some degree of home care has been a recognized aspect of health delivery wherever public concern for health has been generally discussed. However, the historical aspect of home care is not the focus here. This discussion focusses instead on recent developments which have emphasized the need to shift from institutional care to a greater emphasis on home care.

This shift is reflected, for example, in the revival of the Health Centre concept over the last fifteen years. Prior to this it had developed very

little since it was first proposed in The Dawson Report,[28] sixty years ago.
In England the number of health centres rose from 122 in 1969 to 731 in
1977 and whereas in 1969 only 3% of family doctors practised in them by
1977 this had risen to 17%.[29] Further evidence of the shift towards home
care has been the closure of many hospital wards for many of the mentally
ill and some movement away from residential care for the elderly. More
recently there has been the emphasis on the role of the hospital as one for
acute episodes complementing longer term care in the home.

One of the questions that concerns the district nurse and any other
health practitioner is the extent to which the recent emphasis on home
care is genuinely directed towards more appropriate care of at least
similar quality. Graham Woods cites a study in Scotland where it was
estimated that a quarter of those discharged seriously deteriorated within
three months, where the deterioration could be attributed as much to
preventable factors as to unavoidable disease processes.[30] There has been
continual anxiety that the lip service paid to home care may be little more
than a device for saving money on hospital services.

Something of this anxiety was expressed in 1961 when the Minister of
Health, Enoch Powell, proposed reducing the number of mental hospital beds by half within fifteen years. In reply Professor Titmuss asked for
an assurance that money would be earmarked to provide for development of facilities for those transferred in the community so that care is
not being shifted from '. . . trained staff to untrained or ill-equipped staff
or no staff at all'.[31]

While the Health Service might wish to transfer the emphasis to home
care, it experienced the difficulty referred to in the previous section that
much home care provision came under the aegis of the local authorities,
whose priorities and resources might not facilitate the transfer. Local
authorities indeed were somewhat alarmed by the responsibilities which
they were being asked to accept.

A good deal of literature has been critical of institutional care. Fore-
most are authors such as Goffman who wrote an influential study called
Asylums[32] and Townsend who studied Old Peoples Homes and whose
account in *The Last Refuge* made a considerable impact.[33]

The question that remained was whether home care would correct all
the faults attributable to institutional care.

Reliance on the family

Home care is heavily reliant on family or the support of an effective social
network. This must be demonstrably effective and not mere wishful

thinking. Strong, in his study of paediatric medical interviews,[34] noted a strong reluctance on the part of medical personnel to consider the mother as anything but responsible and adequate. The danger is that the family, and nowadays the community, can be misleadingly idealized. Yet unhappily neglect and misery can be the lot of those dependent on an unsympathetic or uncaring family. The difference between neglect in an institution and that in the home is that in the former it may be more visible and more easily controlled.

Modern society has seen an increase in the number of families significantly relying on a member going out to work either part-time or full-time. In this context not only does the cost of a dependent relative decrease their resources, but they lose the income and benefits of work. Thus a good deal of resentment and hostility can be generated in a family where care of a dependent relative has to be accepted. This point is developed by an article by Jane Taylor, *Hidden Labour and the National Health Service*.[35] Idris Williams[36] strikingly refers to the problem of the 'captive spouse' where all social contact is broken for the spouse, burdened with the full-time care of the other. The threat to the home-carer's health has to be taken into account.

If these objections are to be countered there would need to be evidence of a considerable transfer of resources to support adequate levels of home care.

Benefits for the disabled

Improvements have been made in the provision of non-contributory benefits for the disabled. These include the attendance allowance where frequent attention is required by night or day. There is also the non-contributory invalidity pension for those under pensionable age and incapable of work. There is the more generous Mobility Allowance and the Invalid Care Allowance for those of working age who have to stay at home to care for a severely disabled relative. Families with handicapped children may receive some assistance from the Joseph Rowntree Memorial Trust's 'Family Fund'. For those on Supplementary Benefits there may be additions for heating, clothing, laundry or special diets. However, little of it is generous, and none is integrated or comprehensive.

Development of the Primary Health Care Team

Another move towards more effective home care has been the development of the Primary Health Care Team and the expansion in the provision of Health Centres and Group Practices. The primary health care concept was a recognition of the fact that the varied needs of a patient required the skills of a variety of practitioners. Yet to be effective the contribution of each needed to be made in relation to a carefully integrated whole. It is here that the assessment skills of the district nurse are essential for the adequate provision of home care. The development of primary health care teams has been aided by the attachment of district nurses, health visitors and sometimes social workers as well as the provision of ancillary workers to general practices or health centres. Even where attachment is not the prevalent mode good examples of liaison can be found.

Problems exist, however, in getting the different professionals to appreciate and understand each others' competencies and in establishing adequate working relationships. Given this it is perhaps understandable that a system of effective and integrated record-keeping and team reporting is still not adequate.

Health centres do have the advantage of bringing the relevant team members into proximity. Like group practices they encourage the family doctors to keep abreast of developments by contact with one another and other professionals. It encourages the doctors to introduce more resources and equipment as well as permitting a degree of specialization. It also means that he can provide a full service without sacrificing his own proper leisure.

The problems that apply to teams in the management sector discussed in the previous section apply no less to the Primary Health Care Team.

THE COST OF HOME CARE

Adequate home care should not necessarily be cheaper than hospital care. The fact that it is may be attributed to the reliance on the free labour of relatives and the less costly, though by no means less significant, labour costs of primary health care teams. The costs of non-Family Practitioner health services in the year 1976 to 1977 for those of 75 years and over was £365, whereas for those using the Family Practitioner Committee Services it was £60 for a comparable group.[37] Obviously these figures have to be approached with considerable caution, but it does suggest that home care provision could be increased with very likely benefit. Hospital Services in the period from 1968 to 1977 achieved relatively better resource provision than did Community Health Services over the same period. In 1970 hospital services received 65.2% of NHS expenditure in the United Kingdom and in 1977 62.9%. In 1970 Community Health Services received 7.1% of NHS resources and in 1977

6.1%. Allowance has to be made for the changes brought about by the 1974 reorganization. Nevertheless, the development of Community Health Services is a little less than impressive. Community Health Nurses increased from 23 486 in 1971 to 30 937 in 1977 whereas Hospital Nursing Staff increased from 232 636 in 1971 to 286 047 in 1977. Thus while the Community Nurse provision increased at a slightly improved rate it was not substantial.[39] In the same period Hospital Medical Staff increased from 666 971 to 784 440 while General Practitioners increased from 20 597 to 22 327.[40] In the context of an increasingly elderly population and an increasing emphasis on home care it is somewhat disappointing. These figures it must be stressed only indicate a discrepancy in the relative growth of community and hospital staff. An adequate statistical comparison would need a far more sophisticated analysis.

WELFARE PROVISIONS

Much of the support for the sick at home depends on Local Authority welfare provision. This includes the provision of home helps, meals-on-wheels, luncheon clubs, day centres, laundry services, heating and dietary assistance, rehabilitation aids and appliances, telephone provision, holidays and home adaptations.

In the case of local authority provision and provision by voluntary agencies subsidized by local authorities, there is anxiety about the imposition of expenditure cuts. These vary in extent as do the provision of resources by different authorities. Not infrequently cuts are imposed on these already limited provisions. The reduction of places in old peoples homes, the cutting of holidays, charging for meals, the closure of day centres, all lead to more limited home care provision and a greater burden on the home patient and those who care for them. Anxiety about the implications of such measures led to a conference being held in January, 1980, where participants pledged themselves to defend the *Chronically Sick and Disabled Persons Act*, 1970. The conference emphasized the legal obligation of councils to provide according to need, so that where facilities were withdrawn on expenditure grounds action could be taken to question the legality of such withdrawal. In a report from the Ombudsman Sir Idwal Pugh on May 19th, 1976, it was stated that '. . . the Department (of Health) received legal advice that a local authority could not plead lack of money as a reason for not meeting need'.[41] Once again this shows the potential significance of a district nurse's assessment.

An adequate home care system has not yet been established. Indeed it might be said that in the transfer of emphasis from hospital to home, Florence Nightingale's injunction to hospitals 'that they should do the sick no harm' must now be applied to the delivery of home care.

THE CONSUMER'S VOICE

It is first necessary to establish whether the consumer does have a voice. There must be many district nurses and general practitioners who would assure the enquirer that consumers not only have one but are not slow in exercising it. Of course every time a patient pours the medicine down the sink or decides not to bother the nurse or chats to the neighbour about whether she has a 'good nurse' or one who is 'not very nice' they could be said to have a not ineffective voice. It may, or may not be, a very informed voice; either way it may have something to say to the nurse so that she may decide to mend her ways or mend the patient's. It is well known that nurses and doctors like policemen are wonderful. This may be pleasant to hear but naïve to believe. It may also result in a complacency which may not be in the patient's best interest. Patients uncertain of a hearing from their medical practitioners turn to friends, colleagues, neighbours, relatives and sometimes exchange pills as readily as advice. Certainly they have views when pressed about the way they get treated, about the arrangements that are made for consultations, about the difficulty of explaining their problems. They agonise over whether to call out the practitioner at the weekend. If they do not, and the patient needs treatment urgently, they may be taken to task. If they do, and the doctor does not consider it necessary, then again they may find themselves in trouble. The patient is expected to be a good diagnostician at one moment and in the next to passively accept the practitioner's advice.

There may also be a considerable therapeutic value in encouraging the patients or their 'care-giver's voice.' Skipper and Leonard[42] in their study of children being admitted to hospital for tonsillectomy indicate that this is the case. Mothers were positively encouraged to raise their anxieties which to routine hardened staff could easily have been dismissed as 'trivia'. This, Skipper and Leonard suggest, allowed the 'work of worrying to take place'.[43] The consequent reduction in tension seems to have meant that maternal anxiety was not transmitted to the child. The result was a significantly improved outcome in children whose mothers had been encouraged to talk. While studies of district nurses are unfortunately few, it would not perhaps be unreasonable to suggest that allowing patients and their families to express their anxieties and respond to them might well remove a significant source of stress, as well as providing necessary assessment material. It might also provide the opportunity to offer some 'caring education'.

This it might be agreed is commendable, and the district nurse might be encouraged to develop an appropriate technique for encouraging the patient to voice her concerns. Such an activity would have to be accepted as part of her *'real'* work. May Clarke in her research into a chronic mental ward,[44] found that although staff paid due homage to the idea of listening and talking to patients, in unreflective practice they equated the activity with such 'non-serious' activities as staff meals and tea breaks. Real work was lifting, washing and cleaning.

If consideration is moved from the individual patient to the primary health care team it might be asked whether there is a place for the consumer voice. If the view is taken that the patient is a passive recipient of professional care then there is little need to register the consumer voice. Patients should perhaps like children be seen and not heard. If, on the other hand, one accepts that a good deal of home care involves self-management, or management by relatives and furthermore that professional intervention should be appropriate to the circumstances of the case, then perhaps the 'home care-givers' and recipients of care should be heard. Even if it might be inappropriate for the patient or relative to be involved in a case conference, a careful input from the home network should have been obtained.

Again, since the delivery of home care involves considerable administrative arrangements and personnel decisions, might not the patient group, or groups, have an interest in what such arrangements involve. This would require the sensitive handling and perseverance that a fragile hothouse plant requires if it is to be worthwhile. Token participation, a 'friends of the surgery' coffee party for joiners, while decorative is hardly substantial. It would require some hardy and imaginative practitioners to pilot such a project. Tentative beginnings have however been made in some districts with a variety of approaches in developing 'Patient Participation Groups'.[45] These groups may make decision-making slow and difficult because somebody raises objections, yet such is one of the hard facts of a democratic system. It seems a dubious reason for altogether avoiding it.

It could be argued that the need for such an innovation at Health Centre or practice level is unnecessary since there is an already established outlet for the consumer's voice in the Community Health Council. Community Health Councils were set up under the 1973 National Health

Service Reorganization Act. Membership of these health councils is made up of eighteen to thirty people. Half of them are nominated by the Local Authority, a third by voluntary organizations and the rest by the Regional Health Authority. They have the right to be supplied with information and the right to visit health service premises. They have also to be consulted by the Health Authority concerning the effectiveness of provisions, planning and changes in service; they also act as the 'patients friend'.

Unfortunately, their position too often reflects the allegation that they were established as a polite afterthought in the restructuring of the National Health Service. Their role is purely advisory. Their effectiveness is rather dependent on the goodwill of management, which in itself may be sufficient to render them ineffective. There are also problems about their legitimacy in claiming to represent the consumer since very few consumers seem to be aware of their existence. Different Councils have certainly developed their roles very differently. It has been argued that considering their disadvantaged position they have often been surprisingly effective. Nevertheless it would seem reasonable to argue that they need stronger powers to intervene if they are to be more consistently effective. It could be as Klein and Lewis[46] state that a different mode of representation could be devised. It may be that broader based consumer councils should be established. Perhaps as suggested earlier the Health Service could be made responsive by giving Local Authorities control of it. Perhaps Patient Participation Groups might be more effective in the smaller units of District Health Authorities. Whatever the mode the consumer's voice is still relatively feeble and if the patient view is to be effectively expressed needs strengthening. It seems ironical that in a document entitled *Patients First* the value of the Community Health Council is questioned on grounds of cost and the view is taken that management will know best since the new District Health Authorities will be more closely in touch with the needs of the community. However it contains no suggestion about how the District Health Authority can be required to listen to the consumer's voice.

Finally, this section would not be complete if mention was not made of the aggrieved patients voice. Understandably such a voice is not popular since it is probable that it is questioning competence. Such questioning does not accord well with the loyalties of the professional fraternity.

The Health Services Commissioner

One significant contribution to providing the consumer with a voice that would not fall on deaf ears was the establishment, in 1973, of the post of Health Services Commissioner. His field of enquiry is, however, very limited. He is excluded from matters of clinical judgements or challenging the decisions of Family Practitioner Committees. Attempts to broaden his activities to include these areas have met with little success.

The Davies Committee Report[47] suggested that many complaints could have been dealt with by better communications, however, the remainder deserved better formal procedures. Recourse to law, which is available, is both deterrently expensive and not what many patients want. Watkins[48] points out that often what they want is an assurance that procedures will be amended to ensure that someone else does not suffer from the same mistakes. The Davies Report and subsequent recommendations for improved procedures have, for the most part, received an unfavourable reception from the medical profession. Yet as Brown[49] pointed out in his discussion of the difficulties complainants had of achieving a favourable outcome at Disciplinary Committee proceedings 'It is hard to accept that any service performed by human beings can be so immune from criticism.'

REFERENCES

1. National Health Service Reorganization Act, 1973. London: HMSO.
2. *Royal Commission on the National Health Service* (1979) Command 7615 (Merrison Report). London: HMSO.
3. DHSS (1979). *Patients First*. London: HMSO.
4. The Health Service Act, 1980. London: HMSO
5. DHSS (1979). *Patients First*. London: HMSO.
6. National Health Service Act, 1977. London: HMSO.
7. Royal Commission on the National Health Service (1979). (Merrison Report). London: HMSO.
8. DHSS (1979). *Patients First*. London: HMSO.
9. Management Arrangements for the Reorganized National Health Service (1972). London: HMSO.
10. DHSS (1970). The Future Structure of the National Health Service. London: HMSO.
11. *The Times*, 24th January, 1980.
12. DHSS (1972). Management Arrangements for the Reorganised National Health Service (the grey book) para 1, p. 15. London: HMSO.
13. DHSS (1979). *Patients First*. London: HMSO.
14. Royal Commission on the National Health Service. (1979). (Merrison Report) para 20, p. 57). London: HMSO.
15. TITMUSS, R.M. (1974). *Social Policy*, pp. 23–24. London: George Allen & Unwin.
16. COCHRANE, A. (1973). *Effectiveness and Efficiency in the National Health Service*. The Nuffield Provincial Hospitals Trust.
17. McKEOWN, T. (1976). *The Role of Medicine in Society: Dream, Mirage or Nemesis*. Nuffield Provincial Hospital.

18. DHSS. Resource Allocation Working Party (1976). *Sharing Resources for Health in England*. London: HMSO.

19. DHSS Resource Allocation Working Party. (1976). para. 1, p. 3. Quoted in Carrier, J, Brown, M. & Baldwin, S. (1977). *Positive discrimination in the allocation of NHS resources*. In: The Year Book of Social Policy in Britain 1977, RKP 1978.

20. *The Times*, 12th December 1979.

21. DHSS. Health Circular HC (80)8, para. 19. London: DHSS.

22. Royal Commission on the National Health Service (1979). (Merrison Report, para. 16, p. 16). London: HMSO.

23. Royal Commission on the National Health Service. (1979). (Merrison Report, para. 12, p. 38). London: HMSO.

24. Royal Commission on the National Health Service. (1979). (Merrison Report, para. 12, p. 40). London: HMSO.

25. McINTOSH, J. & DINGWALL, R. (1978). Teamwork in theory and practice. In: McIntosh, J. & Dingwall, R. *Readings in the Sociology of Nursing*. London: Churchill Livingstone.

26. STEIN, L. The Doctor Nurse Game. In: Folta, J. & Deck, E. (1979) *A Sociological Framework for Patient Care*, 2nd ed. Sussex: John Wiley.

27. BREARLEY, P., MILES, A., TOPLIS, E., WOODS, G. & GIBBONS, J. (1978). *The Social Context of Health Care*. Oxford: Blackwell.

28. Ministry of Health Consultative Council on Medical and Allied Services. *Interim Report of the Consultative Council on Future Provision of Medical and Allied Services*. (1920). Command 693 (The Dawson Report). London: HMSO.

29. OHE (1979). *Compendium of Health Statistics*. (3rd ed.).

30. WOODS, G. (1978). In: Brearley, P., Gibbon, J., (1978). *The Social Context of Health Care*, Oxford: Blackwell.

31. TITMUSS, R.M. (1968). *Commitment to Welfare*. London: George Allen & Unwin.

32. GOFFMAN, E. (1961). *Asylums*. Harmondsworth: Penguin.

33. TOWNSEND, P. (1962). *The Last Refuge*.

34. STRONG, P.M. (1979). *The Ceremonial Order of the Clinic, Parents, Doctors and Medical Bureaucracy*. London: RKP.

35. TAYLOR, J. (1979). Hidden Labour and the National Health Service. In: *Prospects for the National Health Service*. Atkinson, P., Dingwall, R. & Murcott, A. London: Croom Helm.

36. WILLIAMS, I. (1979). *The Care of the Elderly in the Community*. London: Croom Helm.

37. OHE (1979). *Compendium of Health Statistics*. (3rd ed.), Section 1, p. 1.

38. OHE (1979). *Compendium of Health Statistics*. (3rd ed.), Figure 1, p. 9.

39. OHE (1979). *Compendium of Health Statistics*. (3rd ed.), Table 2, p. 1(b).

40. OHE (1979). *Compendium of Health Statistics*. (3rd ed.), Table 2, p. 1(a).

41. MORRIS, A. *Homicidal Cuts*. Sunday Times 3rd February, 1980.

42. SKIPPER, J.K. & LEONARD, R.C. (1978). *Children, stress and hospitalisation*. In: *Basic Readings in Medical Sociology*, ed. Tuckett, D. & Kauffert, J.M. London: Tavistock.

43. SKIPPER, J.K. & LEONARD, R.C. (1978). *Children, stress and hospitalisation*. In: *Basic Readings in Medical Sociology*, ed. Tuckett, D. & Kauffert, J.M. London: Tavistock.

44. CLARKE, M. (1978). *Getting through the work*. In: *Readings in the Sociology of Nursing*, ed. Dingwall, R. & McIntosh, J. Edinburgh: Churchill Livingstone.

45. PRITCHARD, P. (1979). *Patient participation in Primary Health Care*. In: DHSS *Health Trends* November 1979.

46. KLEIN, R. & LEWIS, J. (1976). *The Politics of Consumer Representation*. Centre for Studies in Social Policy.

47. Report of the Committee on Hospital Complaints Procedure, 1973 (Davies Committee Report). London: DHSS/HMSO.

48. WATKINS, Brian (1978) *The National Health Service: The First Phase 1949-1974 and After*. London: George Allen & Unwin.

49. BROWN, R.G.S. (1978). *The Changing National Health Service*, 2nd ed., London: RKP.

CHAPTER 9

A Policy Background of Welfare Provision

POPULATION AND DEMOGRAPHY

The population of a country depends on a complex relationship of many different factors. Demographers interested in the problems of population have devised various theoretical models in attempts to encapsulate the most significant elements required to understand population change.

Probably the most well known of such models is that proposed by Thomas Malthus in 1798 in his *Essay on the principles of population*.[1] Apart from what he saw as the decidedly mortifying effects of vice, he predicted that, insufficiently checked by moral restraint, the population would increase until it was curbed by the inadequacy of the food supply to sustain it. He wrote that, 'The power of population is so superior to the power in the earth to produce subsistence for man that premature death must in some shape or other visit the human race.' He cited the reducing possibilities of 'sickly seasons, epidemics, pestilence and plague'. If after such calamities there were still too many people for the available food Malthus warned that 'gigantic, inevitable famine stalks in the rear and with one mighty blow levels the population of the world'. While there are populations in some under-developed countries where such a description might appear applicable, it is generally agreed that such a model is a little too simple for industrial societies. The ability of technology to expand food production allows a much more elastic situation than Malthus would have envisaged. It might of course still be argued that such strategems merely postpone the day of reckoning. The question then arises, is there any model available which will help to clarify the ways in which population trends might develop? First it might help, to identify what the recent trend in England and Wales has been.

It is clear that about the beginning of the nineteenth century the population of England and Wales increased enormously and has con-

tinued to increase ever since. With some variation this seems to have
been the characteristic pattern of other industrialized countries. This
increase has alarmed many people and considerable anxiety has been
expressed. A good deal of debate has developed about the exact causes of
this increase. One of the more interesting explanations has been put
forward by McKeown.[2] He suggests that the pattern we can identify is
primarily the result of a decline in the mortality rate especially among the
young. This increased life expectancy and the additional survivors
slightly increase the birth rate when they reach child bearing age. He
attributes the decline in mortality primarily to environmental improvements, especially improved nutrition.

Nutrition improved because food supplies were increased during the
eighteenth and nineteenth centuries. Subsequent to the improvement in
nutrition there were significant developments in the provision of water
supplies, sanitation and food hygiene, especially, in the latter case, with
regard to milk. This McKeown argues broke the link between malnutrition and the prevalence of infectious diseases. As infectious disease
declined the process was accelerated by the continued reduction in the
risk of exposure.

In western industrialized countries a decline in the birth rate has been
evident for much of the time since the mid-nineteenth century and this is
true for England and Wales. This may be attributable to the development and diffusion of more effective techniques of birth regulation. Yet
the willingness to adopt such measures needs also to be explained. The
decline in birth rates seemed to set in some time after the decline in
mortality rates. This would seem to be the result of the maintenance of a
higher birth rate which is advantageous in the context of high infant and
juvenile mortality and economically productive families. The traditional
larger family comes to be seen as a disadvantage, in the context of
experiencing higher living standards and the limitations it imposes on
women's roles.

Thus improvements initiated by declining mortality rates, are
sustained by declining birth rates. What is experienced as a 'population explosion' may simply be the bulge occasioned by the lag
between the birth rate falling, in line with the fall in mortality, before
they adjust at a lower level. This pattern gives rise to a model of
population movement in industrialized countries known as 'The
Demographic Transition Model'. It is sometimes argued that the population problems of developing countries might be resolved by adopting
policies in line with the practices suggested by such a model; that is to
develop their economies.

One important consequence for district nurses of a population sequence such as that illustrated in the demographic transition model is the shift from a predominantly young population to one dominated numerically by the more elderly. In eras of high mortality and shorter life expectancy the population is continually replenished by the young. This pattern is increasingly reversed as the population bulge works its way through, mortality declines, life expectancy increases and birth rates begin to fall. Obviously a population with a higher proportion of elderly people will increasingly strain and stretch resources directed towards them, unless social policies take such factors into account. Certainly the elderly are the group most characteristically in poverty and if current policies remain unaltered their poverty will become increasingly evident.

One factor that can be significant for changes in the population is the inflow or outflow that results from emigration and immigration. Emigration has been important to Britain in the past because of its colonial history and it significantly contributed to the populations of Australia, Canada, New Zealand and South Africa. Similarly the colonial past of Britain accounts for the place of origin of many more recent immigrants.

Other factors however have influenced immigration. The large Jewish influx at the turn of the century was the result of harassment in Tsarist Russia, while the disturbance of war accounts for the presence of Poles, Ukrainians and other Europeans. Finally, shifts in the economy and the demand for labour affect these figures. Many young Australians and Canadians come to Britain for work and for interest. Currently the Strathclyde Education Authority is recruiting young Americans.[2] In 1978 immigration and emigration were almost in balance at about 190 000 persons each way, which is about three per thousand of the population. Emigration has declined a little more than immigration.[3]

There are of course definitional problems involved in measuring these elements. The Irish, for example, have been moving in and out of the area of the United Kingdom for centuries, but of course during the period of the Union they were not distinguishable on the principle of citizenship. Similarly many Ugandan Asians held British passports. In popular parlance many youngsters who have known no neighbourhood outside of Bristol, Leeds or London are referred to as immigrants. Contrary to popular misconceptions the majority of immigrants into Britain are towards the white end of the spectrum. The total 'black' population was in 1976, 1.75 million or 3.3% of the population. Of these about 40% were born in Britain.[4] Recent projections of the number of persons who in 1991 will have some degree of New Commonwealth and Pakistani ethnic origin is somewhere in the range of $2\frac{3}{4}$ to $3\frac{1}{4}$ millions.[5]

DEMOGRAPHY AND HEALTH

Demographic changes may have noticeable consequences for health and health services. The low proportion of elderly among immigrants is a factor in accounting for the lower demands on average that immigrant groups have made on health and welfare facilities, when compared with the original population. A consequence of the ageing of the population is that annual mortality rates may fluctuate more noticeably, since the elderly, who constituted about 5% of the population and 48% of deaths in 1978, are more susceptible to such uncertain variables as cold spells and flu epidemics. Causes of death in the elderly may also be prejudiced, by a heavy proportion of the elderly in the make-up of the figures. Age-specific mortality figures suggests that at all ages below sixty, the rise in ischaemic heart disease mortality may have ceased.[6] Again with all these national demographic figures it is important to appreciate the county and district level variations that may occur within them. In 1977 the West Country, Sussex, North Yorkshire and North West Lancashire showed a significantly higher ratio of retired to working-age persons than did other parts of England.[7]

In the general population the lowest stillbirth, perinatal and neonatal mortality rates are found for second children of mothers in their twenties or early thirties and are highest for children born illegitimate and for mothers aged 35 and over.[8]

Since 1972 there has been a decline in the number of children born with malformations of the central nervous system. These represent a substantial proportion of very seriously disabled children who make significant demands on the health and welfare services.[9]

Obviously significant variations in mortality may relate to the cause of death. 26.75 thousand males died of lung cancer in 1978 compared to 7.59 females. Here changing patterns of smoking among young girls might in due course affect this ratio. Road Vehicle Accidents account for a greater mortality rate among men than among women.[10]

This section is selective and illustrative. It should have indicated the relevance of demographic data for nursing practice. Such data provides the information for estimating the likely requirements for resources and changing need. It may also indicate the significant population that gives rise to anxiety in terms of special health problems or vulnerability to particular condition. The district nurse who studies relevant publications of the Office of Population Censuses and Surveys will find much that will assist her in identifying the changing patterns of population and disease at a national and county level. She may then be able to relate the characteristics of her case loads to the wider situation. Where there are significant variations she may be able to develop a case for a different distribution of resources to, or within her district.

THE GROWTH OF SOCIAL SERVICES DEPARTMENTS

Social Services Departments are a fairly recent innovation. They were brought into being by the *Social Services Act, 1970*. This does not mean that the functions brought together under the Act do not have their origins deeper in the past. If the strands that comprise the work of a modern department are retraced separately they will be found to originate in the Poor Laws or popular movements of Victorian philanthropy, in local authority services and in the provisions of war-time Britain. Residential provision for the elderly can be variously traced to earlier charitable endowments as well as to the Poor Laws. Some social workers began their careers as medical social workers who were originally termed Almoners. The first almoner was appointed by the Charity Organization Society in 1895 to work in the Royal Free Hospital.[11] Domiciliary support for the elderly infirm was first established under war-time Defence regulations and was an extension of provisions made for mothers during their lying-in period under the terms of the *Maternity and Child Welfare Act, 1918*. There have of course been shifts and additions to provisions so that the links are by no means simple.

In order therefore to give a brief account of the rise of the Social Services Departments it would seem appropriate to outline the arrangements of their constitutive elements prior to 1970.

THE ELDERLY

Concern for the elderly can be traced back at least to the *Elizabethan Poor Law of 1601* and certainly the destitute elderly came within the terms of the *Poor Law Amendment Act of 1834*. Frequently provision was made under the regime of the deterrent workhouse, the shame of which was as much feared as its harshness. It was a considerable relief to many old people when the first old age pensions were introduced in 1906. Flora Thompson gives some indiction of what these tiny pensions meant to the elderly in her book *Lark Rise*. 'At first when they went to the Post Office to draw it tears of gratitude would run down the cheeks of some . . . and there were flowers . . . for the girl who merely handed them the money.'[12]

Voluntary Services were also important though the majority of the incapacitated elderly were cared for by families and neighbours.

The Poor Law was abolished finally by the *National Assistance Act, 1948* and responsibility for the welfare of the elderly was placed with the local authorities. This care was essentially residential. Community welfare for the elderly developed piecemeal and patchily. Day Centres were sometimes provided and services such as meals-on-wheels were started. Welfare departments as such, however, were able to provide little outside of residential care.

In the sixties writers such as Peter Townsend[13] increasingly criticized the deprivations that followed admission into even well run old people's homes and suggested that a range of community based provisions would better meet the needs of the elderly. The increasing number of elderly in the population and the rising costs of residential accommodation further encouraged giving consideration to alternative forms of care. It was not, however, until the *Health Services and Public Health Act, 1968* that a framework for a rather more comprehensive and coordinated approach for the care of the elderly was established.

THE HANDICAPPED AND PHYSICALLY DISABLED

For most of the nineteenth century there was little separate provision for the handicapped or disabled. On the basis of destitution they might reluctantly report to the deterrent workhouse.

Workshops and training centres were set up for discharged, disabled soldier injured in the Boer War and the First World War. The Second World War resulted in a greater proportion of civilian casualties than previous wars and they came to be included in retraining schemes. However, as Topliss[14] points out these schemes were focussed on the less severely disabled. Little was provided for the more seriously incapacitated other than National Assistance and the health services. Educational services were provided for the blind and deaf including limited provision of home teachers.

Although Local Authorities were entitled under the National Assistance Act to provide a greater range of facilities and support, few in fact did. The effort that was made focussed on providing aids and adapting homes. Little was done to attack the family problems of stress, frustration, anxiety and isolation that often accompanies handicap.

The first major definition of the social needs of the handicapped was the white paper on Health and Welfare,[15] which recommended a greater variety of assistance but the implementation of its proposals was fitful and limited.

MENTAL DISABILITY

The conditions for treating the sick, including the mentally ill, in the sick wards of the Poor Law workhouses by unskilled pauper nurses was strongly criticized and resulted in the *Metropolitan Poor Act, 1867*, which provided for care in asylums established for that purpose. Arrangements for the care and disposal of the mentally ill was governed by the *Lunacy Act, 1890*, until the *Mental Health Act, 1959* and subsequent amendments. The 1959 Act encouraged the treatment of the mentally ill to be brought more in line with the ordinary provision of medical treatment.

Local Authorities have been empowered since the *Mental Deficiency Act, 1913* to provide residential care and training centres for the mentally defective, while the *Mental Treatment Act, 1930* allowed voluntary admission for mental treatment.

Under the Lunacy and Mental Treatment Acts after-care was usually undertaken by Duly Authorized Officers. These officers had varied backgrounds and trainings. Generally they learnt from practice and their work emphasized the removal of psychiatric emergencies to hospital. Again work with families was limited.

The *Mental Health Act, 1959* required local authorities to take responsibility for after-care and extend the range of provision in the community. Development was thereafter piecemeal and uncertain while integration between hospitals and local authorities was poor. With more community work and an increase in social work assistance the need for family support became ever more evident. Voluntary bodies set up some pilot schemes but after-care was still largely supervisory and people were returned to the environment in which their problems had arisen, thus increasing the risk of relapse. A few authorities provided clubs and day centres but others provided little.

CHILD CARE

Welfare provision traditionally provided arrangements for orphaned children and they came under the legislation of the Poor Laws. Charity provision was also strongly in evidence as it still is. The Waifs and Strays Society now functions as the Church of England Children's Society, and Dr Barnado's and the Catholic children's homes are other familiar examples.

The *Infant Life Protection Act, 1872* legislated to give some measure of protection to fostered infants and in the late nineteenth century the National Society for the Prevention of Cruelty to Children was given statutory authority to prosecute parents suspected of cruelty to their children.

In the latter part of the nineteenth and earlier part of the twentieth century, residential care was the norm for children who became dependent on the public authority. Inevitably there was a degree of involvement in matters of fostering, adoption and community care and these aspects were subject to piecemeal legislation.

By the 1940s children receiving care could come under one or more authorities including Public Assistance, Education, Health and the Home Office. The Home Office set up the Curtis Committee[16] who recommended the establishment of a unified service. This was implemented under the requirements of *The Childrens Act, 1948*. The Act set up the Children's Departments which became responsible for the care, fostering and adoption of children.

Again, however, there was a neglect of the family context. This was corrected, following the recommendations of the Ingleby Committee,[17] by the *Children and Young Persons Act, 1963* which allowed local authorities to offer 'such advice, guidance and assistance as may promote the welfare of children by diminishing the need to receive children into or keep them in care . . . or bring them before a juvenile court'. Section 1 of the Act further permitted a degree of financial support to be offered to families.

TOWARDS CHANGE IN THE ORGANIZATION OF WELFARE

At the end of the 1960s as Brown[18] points out, and as might be inferred from the earlier discussion of this section, a variety of authorities and a range of different personnel were responsible for services of a basically welfare character. Thus often overlapping services might be discreetly offered by the Health, Welfare and Children's departments of local authorities, as well as by the Education, Housing, Hospitals, Probation and Supplementary Benefits Authorities. Then there were the voluntary agencies which paralleled many of the services. Clearly where intervention was undertaken, there was a risk of confusion and uncertainty as a selection of agencies focussed their several workers on the family and its members. Furthermore as Hall[19] makes clear the rapid expansion of expenditure during the fifties in response to demographic changes and a desire to improve the quality of services, suggested that careful control was required.

Another factor encouraging thoughts of change was the difficulty of rationalizing services and planning, in the light of the uncoordinated and haphazard developments that had occurred. This was intensified by the shift towards community care. Yet another trend that favoured rethinking was the move towards professionalization of various welfare personnel. This encouraged the establishment of a more coherent and advanced training drawing on developments in higher education which offered subjects perceived as appropriate to practice. Marshall[20] also points to the importation of psychotherapeutic casework from the United States of America which was enthusiastically taken up by workers seeking a more sophisticated mode of intervention.

A groundswell was thus rising whose movement was indicated by the reports of committees such as Ingleby,[21] Younghusband,[22] Longford,[23] and Kilbrandon.[24] They orientated thinking towards intervention in the context of the family and towards the need for more effective coordination.

The initial suggestion for a united service seems to have come from the late Professor R.M. Titmuss in a speech at the 1965 Congress of the Royal Society of Health. He favoured '. . . a department of social services . . . which would effectively bring together within one administrative structure all social workers in the employ of a single authority'.[25] Titmuss had the backing of a powerful group and was himself influential. As a result of their efforts and other moves to forward developments in the field of social services a committee was set up in December, 1965 known formally as 'The Committee on Local Authority and Allied Personal Social Services'[26] and more popularly as The Seebohm Committee after its chairman, Sir Frederic Seebohm.

The Seebohm Report

Various ways of organizing these personal social services could have been recommended by the Committee. Health Service Groups generally favoured modified or minimal changes to existing arrangements but with strong links to the Health Service. The Queen's Institute of District Nursing wanted the teams already established under general practitioners to be developed further. However the health services were distracted by developments towards reorganizing the National Health Services, just as the local authorities were preoccupied with moves towards their own reorganization. Whatever the reasons, the final report favoured the views of Professor Titmuss and those supported by the generality of social workers.

The report was presented in July 1978. It recommended a new local authority department 'providing a community based and family oriented service . . . available to all'.[27] The department's work was to include the services hitherto 'provided by children's departments, the Welfare Services provided under the *National Assistance Act, 1948*, educational, welfare and child guidance services, the home help service, mental health social work services, other social work services provided by health departments, day nurseries, and certain social welfare works currently undertaken by some housing departments'.[28] Moreover to ensure that the family received a coordinated service the social worker was to be generically trained. This required a training in the skills required for dealing with all forms of intervention undertaken by the department. With some modifications, such as the education service retaining control over some services, the reports proposals were effected by the *Local Authority Social Services Act, 1970*.

SUBSEQUENT DEVELOPMENTS

With the establishment of a Social Services Department a vehicle was created by which further welfare provision could be delivered. As the shift from institutional to community care developed, Social Services Departments frequently had to take the responsibility for providing supportive services. Further expansion resulted from Local Authority reorganization and the identification by the new Department of previously unidentified areas of need.

Social Services Departments are still in their neonatal period. They have not yet totally defined their appropriate territories, satisfactorily ordered their priorities or altogether established the most satisfactory core of knowledge and skills for appropriate intervention. Much of this has to be achieved within the uncertain and contentious political environment of the Local Authority. Certainly like district nursing, social work has to develop in close contact with other services, as Dame Eileen Younghusband points out '. . . in many situations interdisciplinary cooperation is essential. This is because the boundary knowledge of any one of them is the central knowledge of another. . .'[29] The district nurse thus needs to be aware of the contribution that the Social Services Departments can make to the well-being of her patient just as the social worker needs to be aware of the work of the district nurse.

LEGISLATION TO PROTECT THE VULNERABLE

There is a sense in which everybody in society is vulnerable, and because of that is protected by the law. Everybody is thus protected against assault, against theft of their property, and against fraud to the extent that laws are framed against such acts. There are categories of people whose circumstances may render them more liable to harmful acts, which endanger their welfare, than is the rest of the population. Thus children who have lost their parents, have lost a powerful source of protection. Similarly people not in full possession of their senses, whether mental or physical, are less able than most to provide for themselves. Others may find themselves more vulnerable because of the prejudice and discrimination directed towards them. Such groups may find that some protection is afforded to them by law. That protection may not always be sufficient and for some groups may not even be there. This section sets out only to indicate some of the vulnerable groups, who have a degree of legal protection. Obviously, for anybody seeking the precise application and specification of the relevant legislation, more authoritative texts or people would need to be consulted.

CHILDREN'S WELFARE

The *Abortion Act, 1967* was intended to be a compromise between protecting mothers and protecting the developing child. The Act therefore restricted abortion to cases where two doctors agree that one of the following conditions apply:

1. The continuation of pregnancy might jeopardize the mother's life.
2. The continuation of pregnancy could be more of a threat to the mother's physical or mental health, or that of any of the children of the family, than if the pregnancy were terminated.
3. There is a substantial risk that the child could be born with a severe physical or mental abnormality.

Children whether legitimate or illegitimate are entitled to financial support from their father. If this finance is not provided, the child's mother may ask a magistrate to serve a summons.

The *Guardianship Act, 1973* makes decisions about a child's upbringing the responsibility of both parents.

The *Matrimonial Causes Act, 1973* allows a court to award custody of a child, where a marriage breaks down, to whichever parent is considered the more suitable for the child. If neither is considered sufficiently suitable then, under section 43 of the Act, an order may be made committing the child to the care of the local authority.

The *Children's Act, 1948, section 1*, imposes a duty on local social services authorities to receive a child into care if he or she is under seventeen and has no evident parent or guardian, or they are so incapacitated that they cannot provide proper care and the welfare of the child is endangered. The local authority will provide for the child's welfare as long as it is required and the child is under eighteen. At any time a parent, guardian or relative may express their desire to take care of a child and if it is consistent with the child's welfare, they may, after due notice, take responsibility for the child.

The *Children's Act, 1948, section 2.1.*, as substituted by the *Children's Act, 1957, section 57* provides grounds for a local authority to assume parental rights. Generally this happens when parents have died, abandon a child or suffer a serious incapacity rendering them unable to care for the child.

Where a child is at risk and its physical or moral protection requires urgent action to remove it to a safe place, the *Children and Young Persons Act, 1969, section 28.2.*, specifies the conditions under which a police officer may detain a child.

Where a child has been the victim of serious offences, such as physical assault, ill-treatment or neglect, then anybody acting, in the opinion of the justices, in the interests of the child, may apply for a place of safety warrant to a justice under *section* 40 of the *Children and Young Persons Act, 1933*.

When a child has been received into care by the local authority, it may be kept in a community or voluntary home, under the *Children's Act, 1948, section 19*, which is controlled and conducted according to the requirements of the *Children and Young Persons Act, 1969*, but more particularly according to the provisions of the *Community Homes Regulations 1972 (S1. 1972 No. 319)*. On the other hand it may be boarded out with foster parents, under the *Boarding-Out of Children Regulations, 1955 (S1. 1955 No. 1377)*. The local authority may visit foster children and inspect the premises where they live.

The *Nurseries and Child-Minders Regulation Act, 1948* as amended by the *Health Services and Public Health Act, 1968, section 60*, requires the local authority to maintain registers of child-minders and premises where children are looked after. This includes play-groups, nurseries and similar groups. The local authority can make certain conditions apply such as inspection, the maximum number of children, qualifications of staff, safety arrangements, eating arrangements, medical supervision and the maintenance of records.

The *Children's Act, 1975, section 3*, requires that duly authorized bodies concerning themselves with adoption matters shall pay proper regard to all the relevant circumstances, including the child's welfare, throughout its childhood and take account of the wishes and feelings of the child. Considerable care also has to be exercised by the local authority in placing children for adoption.

THE MENTALLY DISORDERED

Adults may be regarded as vulnerable in a variety of conditions and their care may come under various legal enactments. One group is the mentally disordered.

Where it is thought that a person suffering from mental disorder is, or has been, ill-treated, neglected or kept otherwise than under proper control, or is living alone and unable to care for himself then under the provisions of *section 133. 1* of the *Mental Health Act, 1959* application may be made to a justice for a place of safety order. The same warrant can be used to gain entry to premises where access has been refused.

Sections 25, 27, 29, 54 of the *Mental Health Act, 1959* variously allow application to be made for admission to hospital of the mentally disabled.

A local authority may provide support in the community for a mentally disordered person. This may be because they are required to do so by a court or as a result of the person's discharge from hospital under the terms of a guardianship order as set out by the *Mental Health Act, 1959*. The guardian has the power that a father of a child under fourteen has. Other powers are granted by the Act and the *Mental Health (Hospital and Guardianship) Regulation, 1960 (S1. 1960 No. 1241)*. This would include the power to decide the persons place of residence and control their correspondence. It requires the guardian to visit the patient and to ensure that the patient is visited by a doctor.

Day Centres for the mentally disordered are set up under the *Mental Health Act, 1959*.

Certain welfare provision is also made under the *Local Authority Social Services Act, 1970*.

THE CHRONICALLY SICK, THE DISABLED AND THE ELDERLY

A wide variety of groups are covered by provisions for the chronically sick, the handicapped and the elderly. Provision for these groups is subject to considerable variation as the form and quantity of the service are often largely discretionary and different authorities identify different needs and respond variously.

The *Chronically Sick and Disabled Persons Act, 1970*, required local authorities to find out the numbers of chronically sick and disabled people in their areas. They were to identify what special services they required and provide them where necessary. They then had to disseminate information about the services they provided. Local authorities variously identified such items as T.V., radio, outings, practical assistance in the home, travelling assistance, home adaptations, telephones, holidays and provision of meals, in their catalogues of need and provision. *Sections 4 to 7* required certain public buildings to be modified to facilitate access and use by handicapped people. *Sections 17 to 19* encouraged the separation of the elderly and children in hospital and residential facilities. Research into mobility and other aids to living were also encouraged by the Act.

The *National Assistance Act, 1948 (Part 111, Section 21)*, sets out the responsibilities of a local authority to provide residential accommodation for the residents of an area who because of age, infirmity or other circumstances are in need of care and attention not otherwise available to them. Under the Act private residential homes have to be registered. *Section 29* of the Act permits provisions designed to promote the welfare of the deaf, dumb or blind as well as other handicapped people. The supportive services permitted by the Act were extended by the *Chronically Sick and Disabled Persons Act, 1970* and *Schedule 8* of the *National Health Service Act, 1977*. *Section 45* of the *Health Services and Public Health Act, 1968* permits an authority subject to the Secretary of State's approval to make provisions for the elderly and this was the basis for much of the provision of 'meals-on-wheels', home helps, safety aids and the like. Wardens for old people's housing schemes, as well as boarding schemes for the elderly, were similarly provided. *Schedule 45.3* of the Act allowed authorities to employ voluntary organizations dedicated to the welfare of the elderly.

WELFARE BENEFITS

Various legislative enactments cover the provision of welfare assistance. The *National Insurance Act, 1965* provides for unemployment benefit up to a year. It also provides sickness benefit up to twenty-eight weeks, as well as the basic retirement pensions and such allowances as those for maternity, widowhood and death. It is also the basic legislation that governs industrial injury and disability including death. Supplementary provision to these benefits is largely covered by the *National Insurance Acts of 1966, 1971, 1972* as well as the adjustments made by almost continuous subsequent legislation.

The *Ministry of Social Security Act, 1966* and *Social Security Act, 1971* and that of *1980* set out the main supplementary benefits for those whose resources fail to meet a minimum level set by Parliament. This may be because their insurance benefits are themselves not sufficient to reach the level, or because they do not qualify for insurance benefits. The Act distinguishes between supplementary pensions for those of pensionable age and supplementary allowances for those who are younger. Supplementary benefit is meant to be the 'safety net' that prevents anyone not in full-time work falling below a determined level of income. In exceptional circumstances additional allowances can be obtained for such things as special diets, extra heating, special laundry. Other exceptional needs such as replacement bedding, household goods and additional heating may sometimes be met.

Where people are so disabled that they need constant attendance, the *National Insurance Act, 1965* provides constant attendance allowance. Those who have to stay at home to provide full-time care for a severely disabled relative who is in receipt of an attendance allowance, may also be entitled to an Invalid Care allowance. Mobility allowances are available to those virtually unable to walk because of a physical handicap.

RACE RELATIONS

Legislation also exists to afford some protection to those who may be unfairly vulnerable because of prejudice against them. *Section 71* of the *Race Relations Act, 1976*, placed a duty on local authorities to promote good race relations by eliminating unlawful discrimination and encouraging equality of opportunity and good relations between persons of different racial groups. The Act allowed special assistance to be provided to meet some of the particular needs of ethnic groups, for example in some sources of education, training and welfare.

Race relations are difficult to arrange by legislation. However as the Runnymede's Trust's 'Review of the Race Relations Act 1976' pointed out while 'the law cannot be fully effective in protecting good relations (it) can serve to demarcate the intolerable'.

EDUCATION, HOUSING, EMPLOYMENT AND UNEMPLOYMENT

EDUCATION

Education has obtained an increasing proportion of state aid and provision, since the first state grant to schools was introduced in 1830. Nowadays the mass of the population receives education, free at the point of delivery, to whatever standard is judged appropriate for the individual. There has been a greater willingness to finance the provision of a general level of education than there has been a variety of other social services. This is not to suggest that the provision of education does not have its contentious aspects. It could hardly not be considered contentious when schooling is seen as a very significant way for locating a person in an occupational route for a lifetime. Since occupation is so closely related to status, reward and life-style in society, then the means to obtain it are often seen as crucial by the parents.

Many of the debates that trouble the educational waters are concerned with the role of education in the social structure.

There is the debate about whether children of equal ability are more likely to be disadvantaged in the educational process if they come from a lower socio-economic background. If this is so, there is further discussion about whether the schools can do anything significant to compensate for the disadvantage.

Business interests and parents express anxieties about whether standards achieved by the schools are sufficient for a good start in the occupations that children enter. It also leads to debates about the most appropriate content of the curriculum and the weighting of subjects. Against this there are those who believe that curricula should be as open and flexible as possible so that the broader educational aims of developing a child's own particular talent in the widest sphere should be realized.

Finally, there are debates about the form of school organization which is most likely to achieve the aims of parents, society, schools, university, industry and various religious and cultural interests.

As soon as these questions have been posed the dilemmas of those concerned with the development of children's education is evident. It also becomes easy to raise a whole series of supplementary questions that these debates set in motion; what for example would be the most appropriate form of educational provision for the handicapped child?

In the space available here it will obviously be only possible to touch upon a few of the issues involved. Nevertheless a start is something worthwhile, if it leads to further thought.

Equal opportunities

A considerable amount of research suggests that it is the case that children of lower socio-economic backgrounds are more likely to be disadvantaged in the educational process than children of the same initial ability from a higher socio-economic background. Indeed Douglas's study 'The Home and School'[30] suggested that as children progressed through primary school the attainment levels of children from different social backgrounds increasingly diverged to the detriment of those from the lower categories. Dale and Griffiths[31] showed how in a Grammar School children of equal ability were subject to persistent disadvantage if they were in lower socio-economic groupings.

An earlier study on Higher Education[32] had shown that overall differences in children within the same ability bands resulted in a significantly greater number of middle class children achieving 'O' levels and 'A' levels and obtaining university places. It further demonstrated that the highest level of educational attainment was achieved by a diminishing proportion of children as one descended the socio-economic scale. Of course I.Q. tests themselves may introduce further distortion because of the cultural bias that may inhere in them. Halsey, Heath and Ridge[33] conclude in their recent study that '. . . the likelihood of a working class boy receiving a selective education in the mid-fifties and sixties was very little different from that of his parents' generation thirty years earlier', and they further point out '. . . class differentials widen at each rung up the educational ladder . . .' and their conclusion in this matter is that over the forty years of their study 'school inequalities of opportunity have been remarkably stable . . .'[34]

The second question posed in the introduction to this section then arises. Can schools compensate to any significant degree for the disadvantages associated with a low socio-economic background? In the United States the schools were seen as the most hopeful means for deprived groups to overcome their disadvantages. A very prestigious piece of research published as The Coleman Report[35] came as something of a shock when it concluded that family background must account for more of the variations in educational outcome than differences between schools. Later in his book *Inequality*, Jencks[36] reasoned that though expenditure on schools could be justified by making schooldays more enjoyable it could not of itself serve to give more equal life chances. Schooling in his book adds up to little more than the icing on an unequally divided cake.

Nevertheless, while the role of the schools may be less significant than some had hoped, more recent studies suggest that schools can make some positive contribution. In a study of twenty-seven inner London schools Rutter and his colleagues[37] found that whilst the schools cannot redress wider social inequalities they can contribute something worthwhile. They concluded that the way a school is organized and the ethos that is engendered can make a difference to educational outcome. Positive outcomes were associated with well-prepared, punctual, class based lessons under positive, encouraging, optimistic teachers who got on well together and operated a benign régime. Other significant factors included a pleasant environment, agreed policies, pupil responsibility, shared pupil–teacher activities, including out of school trips. Rutter and his colleagues demonstrate the extent to which 'schools can be a force for good'.

The debate that has achieved popularity as the eighties begin concerns standards in the schools and the content of the curriculum. This debate is enlivened more by heat than enlightenment and stems to some extent from the policy of reducing selective education and encouraging comprehensive education. A Conservative government interested in reversing this trend proposes introducing a Government's Assisted Places scheme whereby a thin stratum of the brightest children will be given places in private schools. Quite what the evidence would be that will ensure that particular private schools will be more successful for such 'scholarship' children than the schools they would have otherwise attended in the State sector is not made clear. Auriol Stevens[38] in a study of clever children in Comprehensive Schools points out that there is 'no clear evidence' of a fall in standards since comprehensive reorganization. There is she says 'some slight evidence' that the very top grades in academic examinations is a little reduced and firm proof that 'the general performance of all children has risen.' Overall she sees a gain from the introduction of Comprehensive Schools which is partly attributable to the presence of the brighter children.

The content of the curriculum is another problem. Recent ministry proposals advocate the national establishment of a core curriculum of basic subjects with measured proportions of subjects from nearer the periphery. This implies a greater degree of central control than schools and local authorities are accustomed to experiencing. The reality tends to be that the school determines its own curriculum within the limits tolerated by local authority advisers and Her Majesty's Inspectorate. Some of the inadequacies that arise in subjects such as mathematics may be more a result of shortages in mathematics teachers who find more lucrative posts outside of teaching. What the role of Religion, Politics and a variety of other subjects should be will depend on the resources, patterns and orientations of particular schools and localities. Which is superior would seem more a matter of opinion and argument than indisputable 'fiat'.

The matter of educational provision for handicapped children has recently been raised by the publication of the report of the Committee of Enquiry into the Education of Handicapped Children and Young People — The Warnock Report.[39] The general tenor of the report is that the education of handicapped children should be integrated into the mainstream of education rather than distinguished from ordinary education.

Unfortunately the attention they give to the special needs 'of such children' might seem to undermine their own endeavour. Thus it proposes categorizing 'children with learning difficulties' on a scale of mild, moderate and severe and as Robin Richmond[40] points out it would not be long before such children became the 'CLD's' and little may be gained if proper provision for them is not funded. Richmond argues that a more preventive orientation should have been adopted which asks what are the causes of their educational failure. He suggests that such children tend to come from disadvantaged homes and attend disadvantaged schools. That of course brings us back to the discussion with which this section began. That there is less prospect for improvement for this vulnerable group in the currently gloomy economic climate than in earlier times was made clear by the stress the Education Secretary placed on 'the economic situation and the need for restraint' in discussion of the report in the House of Commons.[41]

HOUSING

Most would agree that shelter is a necessity. The form of shelter used to satisfy that demand is very expensive to site, build and maintain. In addition, housing of whatever variety is very important to people as a source of personal, social and cultural satisfaction. With reference to these aspects we might say that houses are also homes. Finally, few can be unaware that the private ownership of housing may also be an important economic asset.

Given that all these elements may fuse in the bricks and mortar of housing, it is easy to see how important the adequate provision of housing is to people. However, what is adequate for one family or person, may be thoroughly unsatisfactory to another. Young students sharing, may enjoy the top flat in a tower block, which is an anathema to the mother with young children. The large house underoccupied by an elderly lady, while physically unsuitable for her, may, because of her familiarity with it and her sentiments with regard to it, be necessary to her psychological wellbeing. Location close to airports or schools, or shops, or work, may be important to some and not to others. The provision of houses to satisfy people's requirements is therefore very difficult, since there is no easy criterion to assess people's needs and allocate resources.

The White Paper of 1971 'Fair Deal for Housing' stated as its policy objective the achievement of 'a decent home for every family at a price within their means'.[42] The difficulty is that the two terms of the proposition may not coincide, what is within their means may not be decent and what is decent may not be within their means.

The standard of fitness set out in *section 4* of the *Housing Act, 1957* for a dwelling states that:

'. . . regard shall be had to its condition in respect of the following matters . . . (a) repair, (b) stability, (c) freedom from damp, (d) natural lighting, (e) ventilation, (f) water supply, (g) drainage and sanitary conveniences, (h) facilities for storage, preparation and cooking of food and for the disposal of waste water: the house shall be deemed to be unfit for habitation if, and only if, it is so far defective in one or more of the said matters that it is not reasonably suitable for occupation in that condition'.[43]

This still leaves wide discretion in actually reaching a decision and an authority with a difficult financial situation may be very reluctant to willingly acknowledge unfitness which will entail expenditure on its part. The 1976 Housing Condition Survey found about 4% of all households in unfit houses, with another 5% in substandard housing. Apart from these structural problems over 4% of households lived in overcrowded conditions.

In view of the long life of houses another difficulty is determining the standards of construction. If an authority seeks to build as many as possible by building as cheaply as possible, then it may be building the slums of the future. If it builds to standards intended to be adequate for a long period ahead then it may not be able to provide sufficient quantity and be criticized for extravagance.

The homeless

For some people the most pressing problem may not be the standard of their dwelling but not having a dwelling that they can use at all. People may be homeless because of serious domestic disputes or violence, repossession by a landlord, compulsory purchase of a property in which they are a tenant or eviction. If the definition of homelessness were extended to include those who reluctantly share accommodation because they cannot obtain premises of their own then the numbers enduring homelessness is increased. Under *section 1* of *The Housing (Homeless Persons) Act, 1977*, a person is considered homeless if she or he has no accommodation which they are entitled to occupy and did not intentionally become homeless. Local authorities are obliged to afford at least temporary accommodation to those who are homeless and in a priority need group. The category of need emphasizes families with children, pregnant women, the elderly, battered wives, the handicapped and young people at risk of financial or sexual exploitation. Penalties exist to discourage anyone from falsely claiming homelessness. The process of establishing homelessness can be upsetting to people as can the quality of some temporary accommodation.

Substandard housing

Substandard housing arises where multi-occupancy develops in unsuitable housing. This may be because there is a shortage of housing, many people cannot gain access to owner-occupied or local authority housing. Competition for land may increase costs, so that in order to be able to afford accommodation larger numbers have to share limited accommodation and facilities. It may be also that the high prices for houses encourages selling property rather than renting it. Some local authorities may house their less qualified tenants in decaying housing, or the urgency of need may pressure some people to accept housing of a standard that others would refuse. There may thus arise dilapidated estates with a bad reputation, that in themselves constitute a housing problem.

House purchase

House building and buying depends largely on the fluctuation of interest rates. The uncertainties of the market discourage major investment and building tends to be only marginal. Public expenditure restrictions may severely curtail local authority building and maintenance. A resolution of the housing problem is thus rendered even more unlikely. The cost of maintenance and the short term income that may be derived, encourages some authorities to sell off council houses. It may be that the better off tenants tend to buy the better endowed houses. The result may be to depress the quality of stock available within the local authority area and increase the proportion of poorer tenants. This can have the demoralizing result of establishing a stigmatized relationship between local authority tenants and local authority housing. If the local authority rebuilds, any gain from selling accruing to the ratepayers may be dissipated by the high cost of new building at less advantageous rates.

Another cause of substandard housing can be the gap that occurs between planning and implementing plans. People caught in such a development area may find it difficult to move. New tenants may not replace the old, and boarded up properties are targets for vandalism, decline and infestation. The elderly tenant may become isolated, afraid and demoralized.

If there were a single housing problem there could perhaps be a coherent policy response. However, as this section has indicated there are many housing problems and a variety of responses. But the situation is complicated by the fact that the problems and policies are intertwined, and movement in one part opens up problems in another part. This is not to suggest that housing policies are unnecessary. District nurses will be well aware of the impact of housing problems on their patients. Housing policies as Levin[44] has urged must be more discriminating. They must also be pursued more vigorously and persistently if the divergence in housing provision between different groups is not to increase.

EMPLOYMENT AND UNEMPLOYMENT

Employment is a crucial factor in the wellbeing of the individual and the family in a modern industrial society. The standard of life, status, prospects for health and sense of identity and security may all significantly depend on it. The obverse, unemployment may mean the erosion of all of them. The cold statistics of redundancies, industrial closures and rising unemployment figures may create very real fears and anxieties. The economic climate at the beginning of the eighties seems discouragingly bleak as the government forecast which suggested that unemployment totals might reach a figure of two millions by 1981 has proved rather conservative.[45] A figure that represents £6 000 000 000 in lost tax and benefit.

Inevitably this has implications for the welfare and health services which will have to take much of the impact of the individuals and their families deteriorating mental, physical, social and financial wellbeing. Unemployment for many of the older working population could well be more than temporary, and as Sinfield[46] points out they may enter retirement impoverished with significantly greater prospects of a near destitute old age. Even if employment prospects improve they are more likely to do so for younger people who are seen as having more to offer.

Certainly this is not to deny the vital importance of employment for the young, anxious to establish themselves in the world. They have a profound need to establish and provide for families in conditions in which they can take a pride. Unemployment can generate disillusionment, bitterness and resentment which can turn to demoralization and a deepseated apathy. Sinfield[47] writes '. . . if one gives any weight to the greater risk of poverty and the psychological impact of prolonged unemployment then one would expect . . . greater disability, morbidity and earlier death.' In a classic study of unemployment in the severe pre-war depression in Germany[48] the authors wrote that in the early months of unemployment '. . . a feeling of irrevocability and hopelessness had a much more paralyzing effect than economic deprivation itself'.

For some groups the threat of unemployment is much more real and persistent than for others, a point made by Mukherjee[49] who wrote that 'no matter how hard the times are, demand does not fall in the market to an extent comparable to the decline which occurs for unskilled labour.' Sinfield calculated that by the end of 1976 general labourers were almost ten times worse off than all other groups. Unemployment among the higher social groups is less because their positions are better protected by friendship and social obligations. Their qualifications make them less easily replaceable at a later date, their conditions of service may make it quite expensive to dismiss them and they are less likely to find themselves unable to sustain the burdens of their work through deteriorating health or strength. Even when unemployed they may be better provided with pension and insurance arrangements. It tends to be the more handicapped who are more likely to be unemployed and find re-employment a problem. It is ironic that those of working age who cannot easily find employment are also those most likely to be stigmatized and harassed as 'scroungers' both by neighbours and official investigations.[50]

Residents in certain inner city areas may also experience higher rates of unemployment than elsewhere. This may be because of the greater competition for jobs from transient young single workers, the temporary short term structure of jobs that this encourages, the limited educational and skill training facilities of the area, the reduced mobility that results from residence in less favoured local authority housing and a reliance on limited public transport provision.[51]

Poor Working Conditions

Even for those in employment there are some sectors employed at unsatisfactorily low wages, working long and irregular hours, often doing repellent or health damaging work. Their working conditions may be demeaning or subject to the rigours of the weather. The work itself may be dreary and uninviting. They may be readily sacked and their ability to work undermined with age. The less skilled worker may find retraining opportunities limited and costly and find in the words of Marsden and Duff[52] that there is 'no invitation to them to consider work as a sphere where ambition, trust, loyalty and honesty (have) any place'. It is perhaps hardly surprising that Berthoud[53] should find that 'the lower the occupation, the greater the dissatisfaction'.

Yet employment prospects at the beginning of the eighties seem remarkably bleak. The problems that this generates are exacerbated by an increasing unwillingness to recognize rates and taxes as a necessary transfer from the more to the less fortunate. There seems to be a retreat from the commitment agreed at the end of the Second World War to a society, where risks were pooled in the event of unemployment by the provision of effective insurance. The other defence of that society is also threatened, by a less than eager intention to maintain employment at the highest level possible.

ECONOMIC POLICIES

On the one hand there are those politicians and economists who favour an emphasis on policies which incline towards only minimal government intervention. Economic objectives should be left to the force of competition and the free operation of the mechanism of the market. The government should only allow money to be issued that is backed by real productive achievements. This approach argues that employment will be maximized when workers accept the going rate for the going job. The disadvantage of this position is that there is little evidence from the past, or from a broad comparison with other countries that it necessarily produces acceptable standards or levels of employment. Unnecessarily high unemployment and unacceptably low wages could result in what might be termed a 'fruit-machine society.'

On the other hand there are those economists and politicians who would focus their policies on the General Theory of J.M. Keynes. They would argue that far from cutting public expenditure it should be increased. This would have the effect of sustaining employment and providing workers with the wages to buy goods that would keep industry going. This kind of activity is like priming the pump, it may get the process going but there must be substantial economic growth if the process is to be sustained.

Something of the same may be said of those who fall back on solutions stemming from an older tradition that recommends barring foreign imports so that home industries will not be undermined by more competitive goods. There may be a case for temporary selective controls whilst the home industry redirects its efforts to more profitable areas or whilst it improves its product but, in a country as dependent on exports as Britain, any significant shift towards protected markets in the long term could only be detrimental to the British economy.

The fundamental problem is a lack of growth in the economy. Unless one is willing to accept declining standards in the quality and expectancy of life there must be a more efficient use of resources and a degree of real economic growth. This will mean the development of profitable export markets and an innovative technology that will enhance the appeal of products in those markets as well as providing the efficient basis for achieving growth. An advertisement for a sophisticated piece of stereo equipment from Japan claimed that 'if other manufacturers seem a little behind' it is because 'they're stepping back in amazement'.[54] Yet a recent extensive study by the Science Policy Research Unit at Sussex University[55] emphasizes the point that technical innovation in most sectors of British industry compares unfavourably with our main competitors.

In the shorter term there has to be a concerted and imaginative effort to encourage economies, efficiency and productive technology as well as a concern for expanding job opportunities rather than apathetically accepting the miseries of unemployment and an unfair distribution of its consequences.

For the district nurse a successful resolution of the employment problem will ensure a future population more able to sustain themselves independently and a greater provision of the facilities and resources she needs to be effective for those who cannot.

ETHNIC MINORITIES AND THEIR HEALTH NEEDS

Diverse ethnic minority groups have settled in Britain at different times. Some have been settled so long and have so integrated with the wider community that they would hardly be considered, or consider themselves, as an ethnic minority group. This would be the case with many Jewish settlers who came from Eastern Europe at the turn of the century. More recently many West Indians have settled in substantial groups. They may well now have children and grandchildren who have been born in Britain. The same may apply to other groups, Chinese and Cypriots, but others may be of more recent origins such as the Vietnamese or have been supplemented by relatives recently arrived from their original country.

Some groups such as the Irish, the Italians and the Chinese may find it relatively easy to adapt, though there may be some difficulty. Others may find it more difficult and encounter more prejudice and discrimination. They may also find the organization and support for such institutions as the family, health, education and housing, so different from that to which they are accustomed, that they do not readily make the best use of facilities offered, or on the other hand, the facilities offered may be inappropriate for those to whom they are offered.

Any professional group or service that is required by its constitution to meet the needs of all of the members of the society in appropriate need, must therefore, take account of the hindrances that may exist to an effective service delivery.

Most health needs are universal though there are specific conditions which threaten health, that have a higher occurrence in some ethnic groups than in the original population.

Rickets

This is certainly not a new disease in Britain but its incidence among the original population is now uncommon. Recently there have been reports of the occurrence of osteomalacia and rickets in Asian women and children. The most appropriate preventive measure is the administration of vitamin drops. The addition of vitamin D to chapati flour and cooking oil is being considered. While those most at risk are the young and mothers during pregnancy and lactation, deficiency can occur among the house-bound for example the elderly or women in purdah who get little sunshine.

Anaemia

This can also be easily treated although its cause and type need to be established.[56]

The district nurse is certainly in a good position to recognize such conditions and certainly to engage in discussions about dietary needs. Obviously a knowledge on her part of the dietary customs of any ethnic community with which she has contact would be necessary.

Among people of African origin, and less commonly among those of Mediterranean or Middle Eastern origin, sickle cell anaemia may occur as an inherited disorder. Both parents have to be carriers for this to happen. It causes tiredness and weakness, makes the sufferer more prone to serious infection and can in itself lead to pain and critical damage. Whilst there is no cure for the condition sufferers should avoid activities and situations which generate an oxygen shortage. They should avoid temperature extremes, maintain a good diet, take folic acid and promptly treat any infections. Certainly their medical practitioners should be advised of its presence.[57]

Mental Illness

There is some evidence to suggest that rates of mental illness may be higher among West Indians and Pakistanis in Britain. Christopher Bagley[58] in his research on the topic suggests that the situation of these groups and the discrimination they experience engenders alienation and stress rendering them more susceptible to mental illness. The solution to this must be to attack the sources of intolerance and prejudice in the majority population. There is also some evidence to suggest that depression among West Indian mothers results in a reduction of interaction with their children. The consequent withdrawal symptoms in the child may then be mistaken for deafness and mental deficiency.[59]

Asian communities appear not to generate high rates of mental illness. This may be because of the highly supportive family networks that counter isolation or it may be partially the reluctance to acknowledge its presence because of a strong sense of stigma attached to such illness by many Asians. Stigma may be attached much more strongly to such diseases as T.B., epilepsy and asthma by some ethnic groups than it is by the indigenous population.

CULTURAL ATTITUDES TO HEALTH

As significant as diseases themselves are the different cultural attitudes to health, disease and health practices that may exist among groups. The lack of facilities and their high cost as well as traditional medicines in their country of origin may mean that a group still strongly related to its original traditions may not so readily turn to the facilities of the health service as the indigenous people.

Doctors and hospitals may be used only as a last resort and they may, therefore, be regarded with fear and anxiety and contact with them avoided. Also their experience and perceptions of publicly provided health facilities at home may make them very suspicious of such services in Britain. Their ideas of propriety and decency may also be different from those current among health personnel which again may result in poor take-up or anxiety and discomfort in medical settings. They may have different ideas about the proper areas of medical and family concern and they may have notions about the appropriateness and strength of displays of emotion and pain that may seem inappropriate or excessive to the nurse who takes for granted the rules of her own cultural background.

The elderly may have particular difficulties. They are more likely not to be able to speak English adequately and they may have far less understanding of English life. They may experience far more unhappiness and disappointment as they do not experience the deference to the elderly that they could have taken for granted in their country of origin. They may also experience a cultural gulf between themselves and their grandchildren. In such circumstances the district nurse who may be involved with elderly patients of a different culture, should expect to take some trouble to appreciate their views and culture so that she will not unwittingly provide a lower standard of sensitivity, respect and care than she would to her indigenous patient.

REFERENCES

1. MALTHUS, T.R. (1971). *Essay on the Principle of Population*. Baltimore: Penguin.
2. McKEOWN, T. (1976). *The Modern Rise of Population*. London: Edward Arnold.
3. Report in *The Guardian*. 10.4.1980.
4. OPCS. HMSO. Migration Analysis Unit. OPCS. International migration: recent trends in the UK. *Population Trends*, 1979. London: OPCS. HMSO.
5. Commission for Racial Equality. *Immigration Fact Sheet 1*. Revised Feby. 1978.
6. OPCS. HMSO. Immigration Statistics Unit. Population of New Commonwealth and Pakistani Ethnic origin; new projections. *Population Trends, 16*. 1979. London: OPCS. HMSO.
7. OPCS. HMSO. Editorial: Population Trends in 1978. *Population Trends, 18*, Winter 1979. London: OPCS. HMSO.
8. OPCS. HMSO. Craig, J. Comparing Counties. *Population Trends, 19*, Spring, 1980. London: OPCS. HMSO.
9. OPCS. HMSO. Macdonald Davies, I. Perinatal and infant deaths: social and biological factors. *Population Trends, 19*, Spring 1980. London: OPCS. HMSO.
10. OPCS. HMSO. Macdonald Davies, I. Perinatal and infant deaths: social and biological factors. *Population Trends, 19*, Spring 1980. London: OPCS. HMSO.
11. SAINSBURY, E. (1977). *The Personal Social Services*. London: Pitman.
12. THOMPSON, F. *Lark Rise*. The Folio Society ed., 1979, p. 95.
13. TOWNSEND, P. (1962). *The Last Refuge*. London: Routledge & Kegan Paul.
14. TOPLISS, E. (1975). *Provision for the Disabled*. Oxford: Basil Blackwell & Martin Robertson.
15. *Health and Welfare: the Development of Community Care*. HMSO, 1963, Cmnd. 1973.
16. The Home Department, Ministry of Health and Ministry of Education. *Report of the Care of the Children Committee* (Curtis Report). HMSO, 1946, Cmnd. 6922.
17. *Report of the Committee on Children and Young Persons* (Ingleby Report). HMSO, 1960, Cmnd. 1191.
18. BROWN, R.G.S. (1975). *The Management of Welfare*. London: Fontana.
19. HALL, P. (1976). *Reforming the Welfare*. London: Heinemann.
20. MARSHALL, T.H. (1975). *Social Policy* (4th ed.). London: Hutchinson.
21. MARSHALL, T.H. (1975). *Social Policy* (4th ed.). London: Hutchinson.
22. *Health and Welfare Services* (Younghusband Report). HMSO, 1959.
23. *Crime: A Challenge to us All* (The Longford Report). Report of a Labour Party Study Group, June, 1964.
24. Scottish Home and Health Department and Scottish Education Department. *Children and Young Persons in Scotland*. (The Kilbrandon Report), April, 1964, Cmnd. 2306.
25. TITMUSS, R.M. quoted in Younghusband, E. (1978). *Social Work in Britain 1950-1975*, Vol. 1. London: George Allen & Unwin.

26. Report of The Committee on Local Authority and Allied Personal Social Services (Seebohm Committee). Cmnd. 3703, July, 1968.
27. Report of The Committee on Local Authority and Allied Personal Social Services (Seebohm Committee). Cmnd. 3703, July, 1968.
28. Report of The Committee on Local Authority and Allied Personal Social Services (Seebohm Committee). Cmnd. 3703, July, 1968.
29. YOUNGHUSBAND, E. The Past is Present. *Community Care*, April 17, 1980.
30. DOUGLAS, J.W.B. (1964). *The Home and the School*. Herts: MacGibbon & Kee.
31. DALE, R. & GRIFFITHS, S. (1965). *Downstream*. London: RKP.
32. *Report of the Committee on Higher Education*. (Robbins Report), HMSO, 1963 (Cmnd. 2154).
33. HALSEY, A.H., HEATH, A.F. & RIDGE, J.M. (1980). *Origins and Destinations*. Oxford:
34. HALSEY, A.H., HEATH, A.F. & RIDGE, J.M. (1980). *Origins and Destinations*. Oxford:
35. COLEMAN, J.S. (1966). *Equality of Educational Opportunity*. Washington: US Government Printing Office.
36. JENCKS, C. (1973). *Inequality*. London: Allan Lane.
37. RUTTER, M., MAUGHAN, B., MORTIMORE, P. & OUSTON. J. (1979). *Fifteen Thousand Hours*. London: Open Books.
38. STEVENS, A. (1980). *Clever Children in Comprehensive Schools*. London: Harper and Row.
39. *Special Educational Needs* (The Warnock Report). HMSO, 1978.
40. RICHMOND, R. Warnock — Found Waiting and Wanting. *Special Education Forward Trends, Vol. 6, No. 3*. 3.9.1979.
41. New Deal for the Handicapped. Report in *The Guardian*, 4.3.1980.
42. *Fair Deal for Housing*. HMSO. Cmnd. 4728. 1971, para. 5, p. 1.
43. The Housing Act, 1957. London: HMSO.
44. LEVIN, P.H. (1976). Discrimination in Housing Policy, article in Jones, K. (1976) *The Year Book of Social Policy*. London: Routledge & Kegan Paul.
45. Report in *The Times*. 27.2.1980.
46. SINFIELD, A. The Social Meaning of Unemployment, article in Jones, K. (1976). *The Year Book of Social Policy in Britain*. London: Routledge & Kegan Paul.
47. SINFIELD, A. The Social Meaning of Unemployment, article in Jones, K. (1976). *The Year Book of Social Policy in Britain*. London: Routledge & Kegan Paul.
48. JAHODA, M., LAZARFELD, P. & ZEISEL, H. (1972). *Marienthal*. London: Tavistock edition.
49. MUKHERJEE, S. *There's Work to be Done: Unemployment and Manpower Policies*. Manpower Services Commission. London: HMSO, quoted Field, F. (1977). *The Conscript Army*. London: Routledge & Kegan Paul.
50. SINFIELD, A. The Social Meaning of Unemployment, article in Jones, K. (1976). *The Year Book of Social Policy in Britain*. London: Routledge & Kegan Paul.
51. BRAMLEY, G. The Inner City Labour Market, article in Jones, C. (1979). *Urban Deprivation and in the Inner City*. London: Croom Helm.
52. MARSDEN, D.E. & DUFF, E. (1975). *Workless*. Harmondsworth: Penguin.
53. BERTHOUD, R. (1976). *The Disadvantage of Inequality*. London: PEP.
54. Hitachi Advertisement. *Radio Times*. 10-16 May, 1980.
55. PAVITT, K. (1980). *Technical Innovation and British Economic Performance*. London: Macmillan.
56. Rickets and Anaemia. *Report of a Commonwealth Institute Conference*. Commission for Racial Equality, 1975. Reprinted 1977.
57. Commission for Racial Equality. (1979). *Sickle Cell Anaemia*. OSCAR/CRE
58. BAGLEY, C. (1975). Sequels of Alienation, article in Glaser, K. (ed.) *Case Studies in Human Rights and Fundamental Relations*, Vol. 2. The Hague Nyoff.
59. PRICE, S. (1976). *Maternity and Child Care*. London: CRE.

CHAPTER 10

Community Health

THE USE OF STATISTICS

Statistics are too easily dismissed with Disraeli's comment that there are 'lies, damned lies and statistics'. The more likely reason for a reluctance to acknowledge the value of statistics among some medical personnel however may well be their traditional commitment to a personal relationship with their patient. This might seem to render concern with numbers immaterial. This would be a somewhat shortsighted view, since an appreciation of concentrations, of outbreaks of a disease for example, may do more to account for a patient's condition than any amount of testing on the individual. It may also encourage preventive measures that will save the individual from becoming a sickness statistic in the first place. Perhaps the last word justifying the use of statistics in the medical field was written more than a century ago by G.H. Farr in the first quarterly return of health statistics where in 1849 he wrote:

'The present arrangement will show how many marry, how many are born and how many died in England and will thus appear in time to enable the public and Legislature to take the indications which the returns may furnish into account in the conduct of affairs.'[1]

The need to take account of demographic changes, the increase or decrease in birth rates, fertility rates and death rates become obvious, when a health service is introduced which aims to put health facilities at the disposal of the whole population in need. It is for example essential to know the size and rate of increase of an elderly population, if adequate planning to ensure an effective distribution of resources, is to be undertaken in time. The role of strategic planning is one that requires the availability of accurate and sufficient data. If the number of very elderly in the population is to rise, what is the balance of residential and community care and what ought it to be? If an optimum balance is decided, are there enough district nurses in the service and training to provide the desired level of service? Is the role of the district nurse best left alone, narrowed or extended? That of course may depend on the other forms of care available and their distribution. Information is needed to decide the most economical and socially desirable distribution.

If appropriate statistical data are routinely gathered, an unsatisfactory distribution of general or specific health facilities may be shown up. It was such an unsatisfactory imbalance of resources resulting in inequalities in resources available to different health regions which led to the recommendations of the recent 'Resource Allocation Working Party' (RAWP).[2] These recommendations were to redistribute resource allocations on new principles that might lead to improved facilities in relatively deprived regions.

Properly collected data may suggest not only unacceptable imbalances between regions but also between different areas of service provision. Thus the data may provoke questions about the relative underprovision afforded to geriatric, community and mental care. This leads to investigating such questions as the status, attractiveness and dominance of some areas of practice. This in turn may lead to examining the values and attitudes promoted in professional training, the career paths and salary structures and the conditions of service in different sectors of health provision.

A further use of statistics for the rational planning of health provision would be to assist in determining the appropriateness of investment in technology, capital equipment or services. If resources are applied blindly the result may easily be waste, duplication and redundancy. Statistical data are essential to good practice.

Adequate patient care depends upon the provision of sufficient appropriate staff. It is of little use to locate an old people's home in an attractive rural setting if the necessary personnel to staff it cannot be recruited or because transport and timing problems create serious attendance problems. The resultant staff scarcities may be the cause of an unacceptable reduction in patient care. Again appropriate data may help avoid such problems.

Statistics are important not only in planning but also in monitoring the effective functioning of the health service and its component parts.

Exceptional peaks or troughs, relative to the normal data, may draw attention to specific difficulties that need remedying. A sudden rise in the accident rate of a specific age group will immediately require investigation. If certain authorities with populations of elderly people that match the general range, admit a much higher proportion to residential accommodation, then explanations may be sought, perhaps suggesting a much greater capacity of residential accommodation or acute problems in domiciliary care or housing provision. The average length of stay in hospital for a specific procedure may show up particular hospitals which considerably exceed the normal limit. Again investigation is indicated and may reveal difficulties about discharging patients back into a community setting or a shortage of some technical facility the use of which helps rapid recovery. A common use of monitoring is to check the overprescribing of expensive drugs. A higher incidence of certain diseases in some groups may be investigated and reveal a non-take up of preventive treatments, such as immunisation or vaccination, either because of misapprehensions or inadequate communications. Changes in infant mortality may only be recognized and acted upon if routine statistics relevant to infant mortality are collected and properly monitored. Young disabled people may be inappropriately accommodated among geriatric patients. If data is not collected that identifies such young patients, then little may be done to improve their position.

Statistics may be gathered in special circumstances to monitor the success of a pilot project or to monitor the outcome of a new technique or the workings of a new hospital or community health facility.

Such relatively small scale operations suggest another use of national and regional statistics. The gathering of national statistics provides a framework or a general picture, within which a more details and enlarged view may be developed of a smaller element. This small scale research may give quality and depth to the larger picture as well as providing a sounder basis for local action.

A recent example of such research was Malcolm Wicks's[3] enquiry into hypothermia. He developed more precise diagnostic tools to identify the incidence of hypothermia among the elderly. He also proposed the means for distinguishing more rigorously between two problems, hypothermia and the elderly who are cold.

The existence of the broader statistical framework may also encourage surveys of patients' attitudes to services, where it is thought that these may account for deviations in the use of services. Kasl and Cobb,[4] for example, found indications that a greater use of preventive services was associated with a more extensive formal education.

Some data may suggest novel links between features. The fact that the place of birth is recorded on death certificates leads to the possibility of analysing death by birthplace. This may suggest certain environmental factors associated with birthplace that may have given rise to features related to mortality.[5]

Statistics may be as valuable at a local level as they are at a national level. The changing demographic patterns at a local level may be very different from the national trends. In a particular locality the elderly population may be declining or increasing much more rapidly than might be the case at national level. People might be moving into or out of an area at rates which do not reflect national trends. This in turn might affect the appropriate patterns of health delivery. The local numbers and distribution of disabled people may require a matching provision of care.

While there are government statistics published for areas as small as an electoral ward, it may be that there are no statistics on a particular topic that concerns a district nurse in, for example, a health centre. In such cases it may be feasible for her to collect her own statistics. She might want to establish a register of people over seventy-five within her practice district or on her GP's lists. Given such information she would have a target group to whom preventive health and locally designed health education programmes could be addressed. These might include advice on accident prevention, strategies for keeping warm at the lowest cost, or advice on special clinics. Such a register could be the basis for designing efficient and effective good neighbours' schemes that might offset problems associated with the withdrawal of domiciliary services. Given such data, the district nurse could be in a position to offer informed advice that could be taken into account in many areas of local decision making. Obviously the district nurse, like anybody else gathering statistics, would need to select the type of data most suited to her needs.

SOCIO-ECONOMIC INFLUENCES

One of the ways in which routine statistics are categorized is related to socio-economic class. There are five sub-divisions under this heading:

I   Professional
II   Employers and Managers
III Intermediate and Junior Non-Manual
III Skilled Manual
IV   Semi-Skilled Manual
V   Unskilled Manual

As there are other ways of categorizing class the categorization listed above is one of those known as The Registrar-General's classification of Socio-Economic Class, as it is under his auspices that the statistics are collected.

It is a matter of concern that a good deal of the medical data categorized on this basis shows a marked tendency for a clear bias in favour of the higher socio-economic classes and against the lower. This is particularly the case in overall figures for mortality and morbidity. While there is generally a modest downward gradient, the figures for socio-economic class V frequently show a sharp exacerbation of unfavourable figures. This divergence will be emphasized in the discussion that follows as it highlights the major problem. The more modest differentials between other groups should be borne in mind however and recognized in further reading. The divergence between the health experiences of the social classes might not be so disturbing if they had shown a tendency to diminish: This is generally not the case. The Royal Commission recognized this point for it commented that '. . . since the establishment of the NHS the position of those in social classes four and five appears to have worsened relative to those in social classes one and two'.[6] This can be seen by examining the different death rates over the period for the 1930s to the more recent figures.

Table 6. Standardized mortality ratios, adult males under 65 years of age

Period	Social Class				
	I	II	III	IV	V
1930–32	90	94	97	102	111
1949–53	86	92	101	104	118
1959–63	76	81	100	103	143
1970–72	77	81	104	114	137

Source: *Registrar General*[7]

The dominant pattern in mortality statistics is illustrated in the infant stillbirth and mortality rates in the first year of life for legitimate children in the period 1957–77. The rates for social class V were double those of social class I. The mortality rates for males aged between one year and fourteen years old, in the year 1970–72, were again twice as many in social class V as in social class I. Men aged between forty-five and forty-nine years old show a mortality rate of 3710 per million in social class I whereas the comparable group in social class V show a rate of 8206 per million.[8] These figures are simply illustrative. Social class V women show similar patterns of disadvantage although the disparities are more moderate than for men. The dominant trend is for a clear gradation in mortality rates to the disadvantage of the lower social classes but especially to the lowest.

Data on occupational related mortality show a similar pattern of serious disadvantage for social class V when compared with social class I. The mortality rate is more than double for social class V in the cases of infective and parasitic diseases, respiratory diseases, diseases of the nervous system and sense organs, diseases of the genito-urinary system, disease of the skin and sutentaneous system and mortality from accident, poisonings and violence. There are some diseases such as cirrhosis of the liver, poliomyelitis, leukemia and breast cancer where a reverse hierarchy is found. This however in no way compensates for the serious disadvantages experienced by socio-economic class V.[9]

The variations by class of mortality patterns are repeated when it comes to examining the illness data given by morbidity statistics. Some indication of social class differences is given by the data of the General Household Survey. The survey data for 1971–72 indicates that 45% of chronic ill health was activity limiting among the professional class compared with 68% for the lowest social class.[10] Similar patterns are evident in the case of acute illness. The data on the forty-five to sixty-four-year-old male age group for 1976 shows eight days of illness restricted activity per year for socio-economic class I, against thirty-one such days for the unskilled manual workers.[11] Again the difference is consistent among different male age groups, though the range varies with age. Women generally show a comparable variance but with a narrower range.[12]

It is one thing to identify such a relationship between the mortality and morbidity rates of different social classes but quite another to isolate causes. The relationship between life experiences and illness is very far from understood. It is of course particularly difficult, where the factors involved and the possible links are both varied and obscure. The factors that are variously identified as likely causes include, possible differences in standards of nutrition, insufficient income, poorer housing, and greater crowding, unemployment, unhealthy and dangerous working conditions and poorer medical care. It may also be that among groups, the coping response to stress may involve greater health hazards such as smoking. There is, in any case, a steep social class gradient in the three major smoking related diseases, lung cancer, bronchitis and ischaemic heart disease with a very much heavier incidence in social class V that has been increasingly diverging from the figures of social class I.[13] Perhaps the best current evidence of the possibility of such research is that published by Brown and his associates.[14] Brown's research examined the relation between stress producing events involving loss of an important integrating enduring element in a woman's life and the onset of depressive illness. The types of loss involved the realization, for example, of a husband's infidelity, or the loss of hope for decent housing at the birth of a child or the loss of an important job. This loss was identified as the life event which, in certain circumstances, would be likely to result in depression. It was found in the study that the lower social class women were four times more likely to experience an affective disorder than higher social class women. The working class women had experienced fewer personal esteem enhancing experiences in life than their higher social class counterparts. The lower social class groups were also less likely to enjoy what appeared to be the social immunization afforded by an active confidante relationship with a man, such as husband or boy friend or some kind of full or part time work. Brown identified three critical variables that were likely to trigger a depressive condition in those who had suffered a loss. These were the lack of the intimate, confiding relationship referred to above, three or more children under fourteen years of age living at home and the loss of a mother before the daughter was eleven years old. These three are more frequently experienced by working class women than by the middle class. Brown tentatively emphasizes how a sense of achievement may be crucial.[15]

Brown's research is not without its critics, nevertheless it indicates the painstaking and detailed analysis that is required to identify the factors that may contribute to the higher morbidity and mortality among lower social groups.

ACCESS TO HEALTH CARE

Given the discrepancy in health outcomes between the social classes the question arises concerning access to health care.

This depends partly on people's own perception of need. There was for example the lady in an American study[16] who emphasized that she could not afford to be ill, a characteristically lower class complaint. In Britain of course medical treatment is not directly charged to the patient, although prescription costs might deter some poorer people. More likely to deter lower income groups are the incidental costs incurred by seeking treatment for ill health. There may be loss of pay for time off to attend the doctor or the hospital. There can also be stricter lower class norms for recognizing a condition as illness requiring treatment. These of course may inhibit working class people rather more than the middle class. Gordon[17] for example found that 'there is an inverse relationship between socio-economic status and the importance of functional or physical incapacity as a factor in identifying someone as sick'. There is also some difficulty in relating health care access and social class since seeking health care is a minority choice. Wadsworth and colleagues[18] make this clear in their study which demonstrates that more than three-quarters of the adult population will experience at least one disease episode in any month but of these only about one third will consult a doctor. Some idea of access to care may however be gained by considering those who do in fact seek treatment.

Evidence relating social class to access to care is sparse and insecure. It is difficult to find adequate measures. There are little reasons for optimism in this field. A recent comprehensive survey by Walters[19] of the evidence available, suggests that the lower social classes are at least marginally disadvantaged. Certainly they are less likely to be able to draw on any advantages offered by private health care. This conforms to earlier suggestions of Titmuss[20] and Cartwright.[21] Where findings are of correspondence or moderate divergence in care available to the different classes, account has to be taken of the higher morbidity and mortality of the working classes.

The uncomfortable conclusion is that there is more than a grain of truth in the proposition put forward by Tudor Hart[22] as the 'inverse care law'. Tudor Hart expressed this 'law' as being 'that the availability of good medical care tends to vary inversely with the need of the population served'.

Role of the district nurse

The district nurse then, aware of the disadvantages of her lowest social class patients, may try to compensate where the opportunity arises. This may be by encouraging flagging family support in some areas of the working class patient's life. Where this is not possible or appropriate it may be by good neighbour schemes or other groups, who may provide various forms of support. It may be that she can identify differential treatment in her own health centre where working class patients may be disadvantaged. It may also be that even in areas where she seems least able to help, such as inadequate housing, crowding and employment problems, she may sometimes find herself in a position to exert influence to improve conditions for her patients. Finally, she may be able to exert her influence sensitively in health education programmes with her patients and their families, that are particularly tailored to their needs.

URBAN DEPRIVATION

In recent years pockets of deterioration have appeared in many cities. The causes of this deterioration are several and the mix that generates it in one area may not be the same in another. Part of the problem is a demographic one. Population has moved out of some old inner city areas. This in itself might not be a problem but in some areas it is the skilled working population that has moved out in greater proportions than others. This has left those unable to move because of limited skills or age. Apart from a frequently held desire to move to outer areas with newer housing, newer schools and a quieter environment, the move has to some extent been an economic necessity.

In some cities traditional industries such as textiles, docking and warehousing, shipbuilding, rail repair and marshalling yards, and a mixture of manufacturing industries, were subject to closure. This seriously affected employment as industry was not replaced, or the new investment was in office development or land speculation. In London especially industry was discouraged by restrictive legislation during the sixties with the intention of helping environmental improvement by separating industry from housing and reducing the inevitable congestion and pollution associated with it. Furthermore, new industry was advantaged by subsidies in development areas, by easier construction, by ease of access from uncongested roads and by easier freightage to the newer, deep water docking areas.

Housing was also easier to find for workers. Where core industries moved or closed, it often meant the closure of associated networks of small subsidiary firms. Under such circumstances those who could, moved. The unskilled, however, were held because there was little demand for their labour and they frequently occupied council property and were unable to negotiate transfers or exchanges. Office accommodation provided employment for commuters and in any case was inaccessible to the unskilled. In London there was a decline of 5.5% in jobs between 1966–71 but this masks a much higher percentage in particular districts. In three South London boroughs manufacturing employment declined by 25% with an overall employment decline of 12.5%.[23]

With the decline of industry much of a district's infrastructure may be reduced. Transport provision is withdrawn, small trade and leisure facilities disappear, public utilities are reduced. Rising land values may encourage the extensive holding of derelict sites.

Unemployment and population decline reduces spending power in an area and, with little prospect of rejuvenation, stores and shops are moved out or close. This leaves at best, small shops that cannot offer the benefits of low costs derived from economies of scale. Shops offering goods beyond necessities also find the returns in such areas too unreliable and close. Professional services decline with the rundown of a district and the removal of its more affluent population. Housing becomes overcrowded as it is subdivided to offer low rents to a poorer population. At the same time money is saved by not undertaking repairs and the private housing stock becomes increasingly delapidated. Compulsory purchase may be undertaken and in the uncertainties of development purchased areas are allowed to become affected by planning blight. This in turn further encourages emigration of those who can afford to go, while those in distressed situations may move in, because of cheap accommodation. Low rate returns may discourage adequate standards of maintenance and investment in public utilities.

All these factors or a particular critical mix of them, may serve to fragment the original community and break kin and neighbourhood networks. In some cities the problems are increased by massive relocation of large sections of the population from the inner city to the urban periphery.

Social problems

The consequences of such an environment can exacerbate the social problems experienced by many residents. Vandalism and delinquency may increase in the unprotected, and decaying properties giving rise to fear and anxiety among elderly residents. Shopping may be both difficult and relatively expensive. Health facilities may not be readily available and local hospitals may have closed as well as surgeries. Overstrained welfare facilities can result in very limited domiciliary services. The break up of kin and neighbour networks may increase the vulnerability of the handicapped and elderly, while among the unemployed there may be little prospect of employment with possible demoralization and family stress. For the children leisure facilities are withdrawn or vandalized, while schools deteriorate and educational standards suffer. The lack of nursery provision and the demands made upon it make it very difficult for many women to supplement or earn a family living and increases the possibility of stress within the family.

Not every inner city area however suffers from all these characteristics. Apart from inner urban areas which are flourishing, those that are 'run-down' manifest a mix of problems that are uneven. Such areas are not always clearly defined, they may imperceptibly merge with neighbouring streets, so that defining the boundaries of such an area may prove to be most difficult. It is also important to remember that there are more people, in seriously disadvantaged circumstances, living outside such areas than in them and many who are not so disadvantaged may live in the inner city area. In discussing the appropriate policies for such areas therefore, it is important to be aware of the statement in the 1977 White Paper 'Policy for the Inner Cities'[24] which argues that 'the precise mix of problems to be dealt with in each city, and the linkages between them, can be identified only by local examination. Action and policies need to be geared to local circumstances'.

It has been suggested that it might be a solution to grass over some areas.[25] In certain areas such a solution might make sense. Nobody however would suggest this as a wholesale solution. There is too much investment in services and utilities for that to make economic sense. It is obviously vital to improve the economics of these areas, but that suggestion in a time of economic recession indicates how discouraging the situation currently is. It is made worse by cutbacks in the activities of local housing authorities. Some authorities transfer resources from their more affluent areas to maintain standards in their poorer areas. The hope in welfare provision might well be through joint planning between health and social services to promote appropriate schemes. The difficulties of coordinating and financing such joint ventures should not however be under-estimated.

RURAL DEPRIVATION

It is not only the urban area that is subject to the problems of a changing economic structure. Some very rural areas are increasingly becoming areas where, for some people in the community, there is a worrying decline in necessary supports. Farming technology improves and agricultural wages remain low. Small rural industries are facing the problems common to small businesses throughout the country. Economics of scale means that village provision tends to be reduced in favour of extending facilities in provincial towns. Thus shops close in favour of bigger town stores, village schools are closed and the bigger centrally located schools take the children. Professional and health services may also centre on the town; travelling libraries may be withdrawn. Wealthier commuters may increasingly replace the traditional community. Post office facilities may be withdrawn, as may be the public transport provision. For many residents these changes may be of little import since they have cars and are oriented to the town for most of their needs. There are those however who, because of age or low incomes, are more isolated in the village. It may be of course that strong kin and neighbour networks provide very substantial support. There are those though who find that the changing social and economic structure of the village has meant that their kin and neighbours have moved elsewhere, leaving them isolated. Shopping is difficult and expensive because of transport difficulties, while hospital and residential visiting has to be limited. Health facilities are also difficult to reach, particularly dental, optical and chiropody services.[26]

Role of the district nurse

The solutions for rural areas of deprivation like those for urban areas depend very much on local conditions and peculiarities. With some 'urban villages' it has been possible to achieve some improvement by building up good neighbour schemes. These may be just as successful, if not more so in a rural situation. Cooperation can be encouraged that may overcome some of the transport difficulties. Some group shopping rotas may be designed as may library book collection. The milkman or other regular caller may be asked to monitor some of their elderly customers. It may be possible to organize the occasional village excursion or celebration that may serve not only the evidently fragile but help bring vitality to the village. In these situations the district nurse needs to be particularly sensitive to her potential as well as her actual patients. She may be a key figure in helping to identify the specific needs of her area and in encouraging the community to become increasingly supportive. She must also be particularly alert to the broad range of her clients' needs and develop and strengthen the links she has with the wider welfare team. It is by using a support network, that it develops strength and this applies in the rural context as much as in the urban one.

ENVIRONMENT AND DISEASE

Scarcity of oil, the search for alternative fuels and the threats of pollution from oil spillage and nuclear waste have underlined the vital and delicate relationship between man and his environment. This relationship is of crucial importance to those concerned with community health.

Water contamination

Historically the link was well illustrated when in 1855 John Snow demonstrated that the victims of a cholera outbreak in Broad Street, Soho could all be linked with water drunk from a particular pump which had been contaminated by a seepage of drain water.[27] Today, more than century later, four fifths of disease in developing countries can be linked to unsatisfactory water supplies and sewage disposal. 1 300 000 000 people are still without a source of pure drinking water.[28]

Water continues to be a potential source of infection as has been demonstrated by recent outbreaks of 'Legionnaire's disease'. Supplies have always to be secured against the poisoning possibilities of agricultural sprays, chemical wastes and other industrial debris. Wherever there is publicly accessible water there is need for vigilance, whether it is directed towards evident threats or the less obvious hazards such as asbestos dust from corroding cladding settling on a school swimming pool. Water and sewage arrangements, which are normally secure, may become vulnerable under the sudden influx of the summer season's tourists and campers.

The minerals and elements carried in suspension in local water supplies may also affect health outcomes. In a study of cancer deaths in a small rural area Allen-Price identified a higher incidence of cancer in those drinking from wells in a highly mineralized strata than those who drank water from non-mineralized strata.[29] Drinking water may be medicated with a view to health improvement as is the case with the somewhat contentious issue of fluoridation. In some soft water areas the use of lead pipes can give very high concentrates of lead.[30]

Atmospheric pollution

This is another environmental hazard to which a population may be subjected. The London 'smog' of 1952 caused a death rate of epidemic proportions. Legislation under various Clean Air Acts contributed to a significant decline in bronchitis and clearly demonstrated the potential of community approaches in preventive medicine.

Concern is again being expressed about new health hazards in the atmosphere. In Britain alone ten thousand tons of lead are discharged into the atmosphere by vehicle exhausts. This may be inhaled or gain entry into the food chain from its deposition on crops. Duggan[31] has argued that young children are particularly susceptible because they have a proportionally higher intake of lead and a greater susceptibility to it. Duggan takes issue with the DHSS (1978) working party's report on lead in the environment which argued that current levels had no deleterious effects on children. Duggan insists that the evidence available suggests that chronic exposure to low levels of environmental lead is associated with poorer concentration and poorer results from intelligence testing. Further research is currently being undertaken.

Current atmospheric pollutants however pale into insignificance when compared with the breathed air pollutant of cigarette smoke. This is a factor of the cultural environment. In Britain 'at least a quarter of men and a twelfth of women who die before they are 65, do so because they smoke'.[32] Perhaps less significant but a feature of cultural environment is the way that random defecation by dogs is tolerated in Britain. Professor Alan Woodruff of the London School of Hygiene and Tropical Medicine[33] has found that 24% of eight hundred soil samples from parks and playing fields showed evidence of Toxocara which can be transmitted to human beings causing sight damage. Paddling pools, sandpits and parks, verges and beaches constitute areas of risk.

Climatic changes

The climatic environment can also affect health and well being particularly in association with other factors. Bull and Morton[34] found a correlation between temperature changes of particular durations and changes in death rates among the elderly from bronchitis, pneumonia and vascular disease. Macfarlane[35] found a correlation between a significant rise in the daily death rate in London and a very cold spell. Among the elderly who have difficulty in maintaining core body temperatures and lack a suitably warm environment, cold weather brings the risk of hypothermia.[36]

Sudden atmospheric cooling in late summer and early winter may induce bronchial asthma, whilst the climate of spring and summer is associated with the triggering of pollen emission and the subsequent increase in hay fever and rhinitis.

Micro climates such as heating ducts and air conditioning may support insects and viruses that result in illness or infestation.

Biological influences

The biological environment of an area may favour the transmission of certain diseases. This is evident where the anopheles mosquito thrives and transmits malaria. Historically a vivid example was the transmission of bubonic plague by rat fleas.

Nutritional influences

The nutritional environment is of course vital. An adequate diet from both the quantitative and qualitative aspects is necessary. Unhappily in many parts of the world such a basic necessity is not available because of war, drought or soil impoverishment.

In western countries the lack of nutrition is not generally a problem. However in association with cultural factors such as limited exercise, a cultural addiction to sugar, the increased dependence on a restricted diet of convenience foods and a tendency to overeat, there is a considerable need to continue nutritional research. Anxiety may be aroused for example by the change-over in many schools from a balanced diet in the school meal to a self-select cafeteria, where children all too frequently opt for large portions of chips and sticky buns.

High levels of alcohol intake are again a social and nutritional combination that accounts for some local disease patterns.

Occupational health

For many workers, some of the more serious health hazards which they encounter, stem from their occupational environment. There is the noise experienced by some airport workers, pile drivers and disco operators. There are dangers from handling or inhaling injurious substances such as fumes from chemical products and sprays, as well as from dust in quarries and mines. Many accidents occur because of fatigue from long working hours and strain or work in badly ventilated, ill-lighted or noisy situations. Other injuries may be sustained because of the dangerous nature of such jobs as oil rig work, diving, scaffolding and fishing.

Accident prevention

Finally, consideration should be given to the domestic environment. Traffic accidents still constitute a serious hazard for all road users but particularly for motor cyclists and children. Street and vehicle design are important measures for reducing accidents and careful road training is of course essential.

In the home children are at risk from scalds, burns, poisoning and other injuries because of their inquisitive, energetic, unpredictable and unconventional behaviour, combined with their immaturity. They test the designs, fittings and habits of a household to the full. For the elderly, falls are a particular hazard since they are less resilient and the consequences are therefore potentially more serious. The domestic hazards for the elderly are stairs, loose and curled rugs, trailing flexes, uneven surfaces, poor lighting, icy, muddy and broken steps and paths. They are also more likely to suffer from defective vision and hearing, infirmity, forgetfulness, inadvertence and poor adjustment to the limitations of age.

IDENTIFYING THE POPULATION AT RISK

An important means of identifying some of the populations at risk may be the routine gathering of statistics. This is done in the case of many occupational injuries, in the case of road accidents, and other types of injury. Statistics of mortality and morbidity at national and regional level permit the rates to be monitored and inacceptable deviations such as a higher incidence of a particular disease may be related to particular groups within the community on the basis of factors such as occupation, age, sex, diet or drug taking.

Cohort studies which follow a group over a long period, simple surveys or small research exercises may identify groups whose particular life style, age, or condition may be linked with particular environmental threats. Thus Wicks' study *Old and Cold*[37] identifies the most likely group to be at risk from hypothermia. Doll and Hill[38] used a cohort study to confirm the association between smoking and lung cancer.

Public Inspectors may identify unsatisfactory environments for food preparation, or in safety facilities in factories or laboratories. Their reports may identify general inadequacies or warn of new threats.

The monitoring of water supplies, waste disposal or smoke emission may lead to the identification of malfunction pollutants or evasions, which threaten the health of users or local residents. Groups at risk from hay fever and allied allergies may be advised to take measures by the monitoring and broadcasting of pollen counts.

Particular patterns of injuries may be identified with particular locations. Pre-school children in the home environment may be readily associated with accident admissions in hospital.

Finally, screening programmes may be established on sample or full scale populations to identify incipient disease factors that may then be used to relate the illness to a particular group or environment.

The role of the district nurse

The district nurse herself develops considerable practice wisdom which makes her sensitive to peculiar environmental hazards in her particular practice area, enabling her to identify patients at risk. She may then take preventive action, or liaise with other primary care personnel. Equally, team discussions may lead to a realization of a new or increasing incidence of some particular disease or health risk.

REFERENCES

1. FARR, William, cf. Susser & Adelstein (eds.) (1975). *Vital Statistics: a Memorial Volume*. London: Scarecrow Press.
2. DHSS. (1976). Resource Allocation Working Party, *Sharing Resources for Health in England*. London: HMSO.
3. WICKS, M. (1978). *Old and Cold*. London: Heinemann.
4. KASL, S. & COBB, S. 'Health Behaviour, Illness Behaviour and Sick Role Behaviour'. *Archives of Environmental Health*, 12, 246.
5. HMSO, OPCS. *Population Trends, 1979*. London: HMSO.
6. HMSO, (1978). *Royal Commission on the National Health Service Report*, Cmnd. 7615. London: HMSO.
7. HMSO. (1978). *Registrar General's Decennial Supplement England and Wales, 1970-72*, p. 174. London: HMSO.
8. HMSO. (1978). *OPCS Mortality Statistics*. London: HMSO.
9. HMSO. (1978). *Occupational Mortality, 1970-72*. London: HMSO.
10. HMSO, *OPCS, General Household Survey*. London: HMSO.
11. HMSO, *OPCS, General Household Survey*. London: HMSO.
12. HMSO, *OPCS, General Household Survey*. London: HMSO.
13. TOWNSEND, J. 'Smoking and Class', *New Society*, 30 March 1978.
14. BROWN, G. NI-BROLCHAIN, M. & HARRIS, P. 'Social Class and Psychiatric disturbance among women in an urban population' *Sociology*, 19, 1975.
15. BROWN, G. 'The Social Causes of Disease', in Tuckett, D. (ed.) (1976). *An Introduction to Medical Sociology*: London: Tavistock.
16. BLOOM, S. (1963). *The Doctor and the Patient*. Russel Sage.
17. GORDON, G. (1966). *Role Theory and Illness: a Sociological Perspective*. Connecticut: Connecticut University Press.
18. WADSWORTH, M.E.J.., BUTTERWORTH, W.J.H. & BLANEY, R. (1971). *Health and Sickness: the Choice of Treatment*. London: Tavistock.
19. WALTERS, V. (1980). *Class Inequality and Health Care*. London: Croom Helm.
20. TITMUSS, R.M. (1968). *Commitment to Welfare*. London: Allen & Unwin.
21. CARTWRIGHT, A. 'What Goes on in the Doctor's Surgery?', art. in Acheson & Aird, *Seminars in Community Medicine*, Vol. 1. Oxford, 1976.
22. TUDOR HART, J. 'The Inverse Care Law', *The Lancet*, Feb. 7, 1971.
23. GRIPAIOS, P. 'The Closure of Firms in the Inner City . . .'. *Regional Studies*, 11. 1977 (p. 1 footnote).
24. HMSO *Policy for the Inner Cities*, Cmd 6845. London: HMSO.
25. DENMAN, D.R. 'Should we put our cities out to grass?' *New Society*, 30 June 1977.
26. SIMPSON, R. (1979). *Access to Primary Care*, Research Paper No. 6. London: HMSO.
27. HOWE, M.G. (1976). *Man, Environment and Disease in Britain*. Harmondsworth: Penguin.
28. BBC Radio Report, 11.11. 1980.
29. ALLEN-PRICE, E.D. 'Uneven Distribution of Cancer in West Devon, *Lancet*, *1*, (1960), quoted in Howe, M.G. (1976). *Man, Environment and Disease in Britain*, p. 58. Harmondsworth: Penguin.
30. DUGGAN, M. *'Futures'*, Report in *The Guardian* (p.15), 6.11.1980.
31. DUGGAN, M. *'Futures'*, Report in *The Guardian* (p.15), 6.11.1980.

32. TOWNSEND, J. 'Smoking and Class', *New Society*, 30 March, 1978.
33. Report, *The Guardian*, 21.5.80.
34. BULL, G.M. & MORTON, J. 'Relationship of Temperature with Death Rates from all Causes and from Certain Respiratory and Arteriosclerotic Diseases in Different Age Groups', *Age and Ageing*. **4**. 232. 1975. Quoted in Wicks, M. *op. cit*. Ch. 10.
35. MACFARLANE, Alison. 'Daily Deaths in Greater London', *Population Trends 5*, HMSO Autumn 1976, p. 24. Quoted in Wicks, M. (1978). *Old and Cold*, Ch. 10.
36. WICKS, M. (1978). *Old and Cold*. London: Heinemann.
37. WICKS, M. (1978). *Old and Cold*. London: Heinemann.
38. DOLL, R. & HILL, A.B. 'Mortality in Relation to Smoking: Ten Years Observations of British Doctors', *Br. med. J.*, **1**. 1399–1400, 1400–1467.

Index